The Role of Emotion and Affe

Nancy McNaughton

The Role of Emotion and Affect in the Work of Standardized Patients

A Theoretical Analysis

LAP LAMBERT Academic Publishing

Impressum / Imprint
Bibliografische Information der Deutschen Nationalbibliothek: Die Deutsche Nationalbibliothek verzeichnet diese Publikation in der Deutschen Nationalbibliografie; detaillierte bibliografische Daten sind im Internet über http://dnb.d-nb.de abrufbar.
Alle in diesem Buch genannten Marken und Produktnamen unterliegen warenzeichen-, marken- oder patentrechtlichem Schutz bzw. sind Warenzeichen oder eingetragene Warenzeichen der jeweiligen Inhaber. Die Wiedergabe von Marken, Produktnamen, Gebrauchsnamen, Handelsnamen, Warenbezeichnungen u.s.w. in diesem Werk berechtigt auch ohne besondere Kennzeichnung nicht zu der Annahme, dass solche Namen im Sinne der Warenzeichen- und Markenschutzgesetzgebung als frei zu betrachten wären und daher von jedermann benutzt werden dürften.

Bibliographic information published by the Deutsche Nationalbibliothek: The Deutsche Nationalbibliothek lists this publication in the Deutsche Nationalbibliografie; detailed bibliographic data are available in the Internet at http://dnb.d-nb.de.
Any brand names and product names mentioned in this book are subject to trademark, brand or patent protection and are trademarks or registered trademarks of their respective holders. The use of brand names, product names, common names, trade names, product descriptions etc. even without a particular marking in this works is in no way to be construed to mean that such names may be regarded as unrestricted in respect of trademark and brand protection legislation and could thus be used by anyone.

Coverbild / Cover image: www.ingimage.com

Verlag / Publisher:
LAP LAMBERT Academic Publishing
ist ein Imprint der / is a trademark of
AV Akademikerverlag GmbH & Co. KG
Heinrich-Böcking-Str. 6-8, 66121 Saarbrücken, Deutschland / Germany
Email: info@lap-publishing.com

Herstellung: siehe letzte Seite /
Printed at: see last page
ISBN: 978-3-659-26257-9

Zugl. / Approved by: Toronto, University of Toronto, Diss., 2012

Copyright © 2012 AV Akademikerverlag GmbH & Co. KG
Alle Rechte vorbehalten. / All rights reserved. Saarbrücken 2012

The Role of Emotion and Affect in the Work of Standardized Patients:

A Critical Theoretical Analysis

Preface

Standardized Patients (SPs) are lay persons who are employed extensively within health professional education to help teach and assess a range of clinical skills. Individuals trained to take on the physical, historical and emotional aspects of patient stories are integral to the dissemination of collective attitudes, values, and beliefs about what it means to be a competent health professional. As an embodied affective presence literally in front of and often in physical contact with health professionals SPs are a fertile site of knowledge production as well as transformative learning. Their unique contribution is a corollary of both their location as non-clinicians and their pedagogical facility with embodied emotions and affect.

SPs in medical education teach about emotion and affect, engage affectively in the presentation of clinical material and as a professionalizing group have developed an educational methodology for facilitating understanding and experience of emotion and affect.

In this thesis I examine the field of human simulation and the work of standardized patients (SPs) through critical theoretical perspectives seeking to broaden our understanding of their contributions as a present and future force in health professional education, specifically medical education. Central to my examination is the constitutive role of emotion and affect as they are conceived both within medical education and engaged by standardized patients as media through which different knowledges are produced.

My analysis is shaped by poststructuralist feminist writers on emotion, Michel Foucault's genealogical historical approach, and principally Gilles

Deleuze and Felix Guattari's alternative nomadology as theorized in *a thousand plateaus* (1987). I intend an alternative reading of the advent of SPs in medical education through a process of mapping rhizomatic networks that include acting, emotion, affect, medicine, and the place of women patients and standardized patients in medical arenas.

I have located the current study within an ongoing project of embodied ethical practice and nomadic subjectivity within education specific to human simulation and standardized patients.

Acknowledgements

I would like first to acknowledge the love and support of my family. Dan, your perfectly timed cups of tea and patience (you never once asked me when I was going to finish), provided me with a safe space in which to thrash around over my many years of writing. Sam and Max your pride in me and your unflagging interest in my work has meant so much to me over the years. I am thrilled to be sharing my thesis with the University of Toronto Standardized Patient Program and the many SPs who have shared their stories with me during frequent philosophical debates about the work that we are all tied to as a tribe. I am grateful to my friends and colleagues from whom I received encouragement, and steadying assistance that sustained me along the way: Kerry Knickle, Diana Tabak, LJ Nelles, Tina Martimianakis, Anja Robb and Rachel Ellis and Brian Simmons.

I am deeply grateful to Brian Hodges my dear friend and mentor who has made the journey both fun and fulfilling as well as Megan Boler whose critical work on emotion started me on this journey and whose deep reading of my thesis served to expand and clarify my thinking and final writing. Finally I am most deeply thankful for Jamie Magnusson, my supervisor and teacher for her patient and grounded commitment to my work and its many semi-coherent iterations. Our relationship truly has been one of following, entailing a close moment to moment listening and respect for what is emerging along the path. Finally I acknowledge my sister who was my longest life companion and fellow traveller with whom I wrangled with Deleuze, Guattari, and Spinoza by way of Nietzsche while also spending hours trying to make sense of Foucault and Artaud. She was a creative force to so many people and I sorely miss her especially now.

Table of Contents

PREFACE II

ACKNOWLEDGEMENTS IV

TABLE OF CONTENTS V

DEDICATION XIII

CHAPTER 1 THE SETTING 1

1.0   Introduction 1

1.1   SPs as Teachers 3

1.2   My Location 6

1.3   The Problem Space 8

    1.3.1   Teaching Emotion as Communication Skill 9

    1.3.2   It begins with a body, my body 12

    1.3.3   Gendering of a field 14

    1.3.4   Teaching Story: Ethics Part I 19

        1.3.4.1   Ethics of representation: Perpetually Possible Patient 22

1.4   Conclusion 24

1.5.   Organization of Thesis 24

CHAPTER 2: THEORETICAL INFLUENCES 28

2.0	Introduction	28
2.1	Affective Mannequin	28
2.2	Theorizing Emotion and Affect	31
2.3.	Theoretical Influences	33
2.3.1	Feminist Post structuralism	33
2.3.2	Foucauldian Contributions	37
2.3.3	Deleuze and Guattari	40
2.3.3.1	Pragmatics: Nomad Thought	41
2.4	Definitions	42
2.4.1	Rhizome	43
2.4.2	Multiplicity	44
2.4.3	Lines Molar, Molecular and Lines of Flight	44
2.4.4	Haecceity	46
2.4.5	Assemblages	47
2.4.6	Desire	48
2.4.7	Royal Societies/Royal Science	50
2.5	Affect and Simulation in Medical Education	50
2.6	Conclusion	52
	Notes	54

CHAPTER 3 AFFECT, EMOTION, STANDARDIZED PATIENTS & MEDICAL EDUCATION 55

3.0 Introduction: Nomadic Ethics 55

3.1 Emotion and Affect in Medical Education 56

3.2 Emotion in Medical Education 58

   3.2.1 Emotion: as Interpersonal Technique 59

   3.2.2 Gender/ Bodies/Emotion and Medical Professionalism 62

3.3 Emotional Intelligence and Medical Education 66

   3.3.1 Models of Emotional intelligence 67

   3.3.2 Emotional Intelligence: Main Ideas 70

   3.3.4 Achieving Emotional Competency 72

   3.3.5 E.I. Models and Measurement 73

   3.3.6 Emotional Intelligence: Products and Practices in Medical Education 74

3.4 Emotion: a problem to be fixed 76

   3.4.1 Emotion as Demonstration of Skill 78

   3.4.2 Implications of an E.I. Assemblage in Medical Education Training 81

3.5 Empathy 82

   3.5.1 Empathy as Detached Concern 83

	3.5.2 Effect on Medical Trainees	84
	3.5.3 Effect on the Medical Professional	86
	3.5.4 Effect on the Patient	88
3.6.	Witnessing: An alternative understanding	91
3.7	Affect	93
	3.7.1 Affect/Expression	95
3.8	Towards a Nomadic Ethics: "So that is how you survive?"	97
3.9	Conclusion	101
	Notes	102

CHAPTER 4 THE FIELD OF MEDICAL SIMULATION: AN OVERVIEW 103

4.0	The Market Place	103
4.1	Introduction	104
4.2	Background	105
4.3	Genealogy of Medical Simulation	106
	4.3.1 From Military to Medicine	108
	4.3.1.2 Military Theatre	109
	4.3.2 Patient Safety and Medical Error Reduction	112
4.4	Medical Simulation	113

- 4.4.1 Fidelity 114
- 4.4.2 Medical Simulation Modalities 116
- 4.4.2.1 Part Task Trainers 116
- 4.5 A Brief History of Mannequins 117
- 4.5.1 Full Body Mannequins 117
- 4.6 Social and Ethical Concerns 119
- 4.7 Virtual and computer based systems 122
- 4.8 Human Cadaver and Animal Models 125
- 4.9 Hybrid Simulation 126
- 4.10 Human Simulation: Fleshy Mannequins 127
- 4.11 Conclusion 131
- Notes 135

CHAPTER 5 HUMAN SIMULATION: A MAPPING 137

- 5.0 Introduction 137
- 5.1 Duplicity/Representation 138
- 5.2 Heather's story 141
- 5.3 Acting and Passion 144
- 5.4 Mapping Passion 146
- 5.5 Acting and Human Simulation 148

5.6   Embodied Emotion and Performance of Illness 151

5.7   Embodied Emotion and Performance of Social Roles 152

5.8   An Anti- Genealogy of Human Simulation: Medicine, Charlatans, Mountebanks and Quacksalvers 153

   5.8.1   SPs /Nomads 155

5.9   Hysteria: A Genealogical mapping 156

5.10 Hysteria and Simulation 159

   5.10.1. Simulating Hysteria 160

   5.10.2   Hysteria as Theatre 162

   5.10.3   Complicity/Performance 164

   5.10.4   Representation/Performance/Simulation/Acting: The Invisible Made Visible 166

   5.10.5   Duplicity/Representation – Complicity/Performance 168

5.11 Conclusion 170

   Notes 173

CHAPTER 6 STANDARDIZED PATIENTS, THE STATE, AND THE NOMAD WAR MACHINE 176

6.0   Introduction 176

6.1   The State and royal science 177

   6.1.1   OSCE training 179

	6.1.2	OSCE and the State	181
6.2		Emotion Affect and Assessment Assemblages	186
6.3		The war machine/nomads	188
	6.3.1	Nomad Space	189
	6.3.2	Nomad Professionals	192
6.4		Becoming Patient	194
	6.4.1	Mary Rice (child abuser)	195
	6.4.2	Preparing for Mary	196
	6.4.3	Enacting Mary	200
	6.4.3.1	Surfaces of Skin, Action and Gesture	205
6.5		Assemblages of Desire: SP-Actor-Nomad	207
6.6		Conclusion	209
		Notes	212

CHAPTER 7 A DELEUZIAN ENACTMENT OF A FOUCAULDIAN SPACE 215

7.0		Introduction	215
7.1		Performance and Pedagogy	215
7.2		Performing the Medical Educational Gaze	217
	7.2.1	Abstract	217

7.2.2		Ethics Performed	218
7.3	The Performance		219
7.3.1		Setting	219
7.3.2		Scene I	219
7.3.2.1		Scene II	230
7.3.2.2		Epilogue I	235
7.3.3		Epilogue II: A dance not a march	236
7.4	Performance		239
7.4.1		Performance as Nomadic ethics	240
7.4.2		Emotion and Affect as Aesthetic Performance	241
7.4.3		SP Performances and Transpositions	243
7.5	Conclusion		245
	Notes		247
CHAPTER 8 FINAL REFLECTIONS			251
8.0	Reflections		251
REFERENCES			254

Dedication

In memory of my sister Susan

andthe miracle of uneventful days

Chapter 1 The Setting

1.0 Introduction

Medicine is a profession constituted by science, social science, arts, and the humanities. Medical education incorporates, with varying degrees of success, ideas from all of these fields to inform its practice. There is a rich literature within medical education covering curriculum design and implementation and the pros and cons of different forms of pedagogy, evaluation and assessment. Historical treatments of medicine as a profession and medical education as a field are also endemic as are debates about professionalism and competency and the educational theories that inform them. Traditionally theorized within positivist frameworks in which inquiry focuses on measurable and generalizable outcomes, these areas are now being examined from critical socio cultural perspectives. A growing number of scholars are currently addressing issues within medical education related to power and the influence of social and cultural theory (Bleakley, 2006, 2011; Bligh, 2006; Good, 2003; Hodges, 2004, 2005, 2006, 2007; Lingard, 2002, 2009; Martimianakis, 2009; Wear, 1997, 2006; 2009 etc.). It is a welcome movement that seeks to broaden our understanding about the ways in which medical education and medicine itself intersect with larger social concerns.

Much of the literature on pedagogy within medical education addresses practical aspects of training and coaching techniques, course design, educational methodologies such as problem based learning (PBL), and the ever expanding simulation technologies, with the focus on knowledge and skills acquisition rather than teacher practices *per se*. A large part of this literature is dedicated to assessment methodologies with particular attention to performance assessments of which there are many forms, the Objective Structured Clinical Examinations (OSCE) being the most well known. Little attention has been paid explicitly to either the role of standardized patients as sites of knowledge production or emotion and affect in medical education. Where emotion is engaged pedagogically it shows up most often as "values" and "attitudes" with a focus on how these might best be transmitted and assessed as a form of "emotional intelligence" or skill. No research to my knowledge has examined the role of emotion and affect in teaching specifically by non clinician teachers such as standardized patients (SPs) or what the work of these educators entails.

I am interested in how taken for granted ideas about emotion and affect in medical training activate professional expectations about emotion and affect in practice and the part standardized patients play in the process. However I am also examining how medical professional expectations have informed the field of human simulation and the teaching work of standardized patents. How do different ideas about emotion and affect intersect with medicine's epistemic authority to produce subject positions such as standardized patients? I will be theorizing about these relationships within critical frameworks in order to understand emotion and affect as part of an ongoing project of ethical practices. This interest stems from my training and work as a professional actor and my many years working in the standardized patient field. From my vantage point emotion is visible as a tangible force in medical training yet is addressed within scientific frameworks which elide it as a valid topic of discussion in the practice of medicine. There is a lacuna between legitimate science and illegitimate art where non clinicians, enacting patient stories' are able to interrupt established truths about the practice of medicine as rational pursuit.

Emotion is constituted as feminine territory in medicine and is put to work through mechanisms that attempt to nail it down, tame it and use it as a tool for professional ends. Acting, emotion and gender intersect in ways that inform my story and the work of standardized patients. In particular I am concerned with making visible the political/professional implications that different ideas about emotion within medical education have on human simulation and the educators who enact it.

1.1 SPs as Teachers

My focus in this thesis is on the teaching work in which SPs and those now identified as SP educators engage. This work entails multiple locations and activities within medical education ranging from portraying an array of roles as part of teaching, to teaching by facilitating other SPs in a role interacting with a student in a clinical encounter. SPs are required to enact anything ranging from an inert body for physical exam skills teaching to a patient suffering from any number of complex emotional and psychological experiences of loss, addiction, mental illness and more. As a *technology* SPs are "used" to teach "about" different topics and may or may not be asked to provide feedback about their experience as the "patient" in their encounters. For example, in a physical exam teaching session the SP's body is the teaching tool, which engages in nonverbal feedback through its responsiveness to the students touch and queries. In other words SPs are always engaged affectively through their work with students, whether they are asked to express their experiences verbally or not. Feedback when it is requested is specifically formulated, and delimited by the objectives of the educational session. Unlike the large range of mannequins and other machinery which are also used for teaching, SPs even at their most lifeless inhabit a teaching space affectively, providing students with often immeasurable experiences through verbal and non verbal feedback. I will elaborate on this idea of teaching as an embodied praxis throughout my thesis. The idea of SPs as a *technology* or tool is supported by and supports practices related to standardization and "...neatly packaged so-called universals claimed as accurate or valid representations [...]" (O'Riley, 2003, p. 62). The notion of SPs as a technology is maintained by many within the field of human simulation extending back to its inception by neurologist Howard Barrows. The question is not whether SPs are or are not tools but rather what kind of technology SPs represent and in relation to whose vision?

The power differential that is created by legitimizing the use of lay people for teaching in the medical academy cannot be ignored. Standardized patients are not "real" patients nor do they represent real patients but rather physician's ideas about specific patient cases. Roles are loosely based on real stories that are then modified for educational purposes. The "patient" is a palimpsest written over by medical educational objectives. There is often no contact between the patient whose story and experience is being enacted and the SP enacting it. Rather SP roles and portrayals are vehicles for the transmission and reproduction of professional values, attitudes, clinical knowledge and skill.SP work is a political and cultural undertaking which crosses borders and facilitates alliances among differently located constituents.

Over many years and in conjunction with changes in societal expectations about physicians' professional responsibilities to communicate with patients differently, and patients' increasing demand for accountability and greater say in their own care, a professionalizing standardized patient group has developed expertise in different domains of clinical knowledge as well as pedagogical and assessment practices. This growing expertise encompasses clinical and non clinical knowledge about the components and organization of interviews, multiple examination techniques, (neurological, respiratory, orthopaedic, etc.) as well as the ability to teach about these alongside the affective elements of a medical interaction from a patient or lay person perspective. These veteran standardized patients identified as educators within the field of medical education engage live simulation as an experiential *methodology*. Like other SPs they may enact roles, provide feedback about their responses, and provide instruction following an encounter through verbal feedback. However, now they also take on the role of facilitator as third party (with another SP in role), either alongside a clinician teacher or alone, for groups of students as well as practicing professionals who are learning through live simulation. This cadre of educators is invited to design curriculum, SP roles, and other educational material and initiatives calling on their expert knowledge of live simulation as both a *technology* and a *methodology*.

Gender is essential to the story of human simulation and standardized patients as teachers. The name for the tool to be used was provided by men; however, the field was developed and is dominated by women. Together, acting, women and medicine form a matrix that informs the shape and possibilities for SP work. This is especially so in formative settings where alternative imaginings of patient experiences are made possible in resistance to objectification by a universalizing "medical education gaze".

I suggest that as teachers, SPs are integral to the dissemination of collective attitudes, and beliefs about what it means to be a health professional. Their unique contribution to students' professional socialization processes is a corollary of both their location as non-clinicians and their pedagogical engagement of emotion and affect. In my experience as an SP, now acting as a teacher and scholar, the teaching includes emotion and affect as embodied performances specific to a given historical and cultural moment and location. "A performative view of emotion focuses on the dynamic process of discursive practices *and* the materiality of the body in various modes of representation" (Zembylas, 2005, p. 35). These are assemblages in which different discourses trouble and reveal subjectivity, agency, resistance, and teaching and learning as contingent sites of knowledge production. An embodied and affective pedagogy views teaching and learning as a landscape of connections. As embodied sites of knowledge production SPs are not passive matter waiting to be shaped but are "desiring machines"[1] through which affective connections create new understandings.

1.2 My Location

> A simulated/standardized patient is a healthy person or one who has "chronic stable" findings and who has been coached to portray the affect and history of an actual patient so accurately that the simulation cannot be detected by a skilled clinician (Barrows, 1987).

I am writing as a standardized patient (SP) and someone who for over twenty six years has worked as a teacher, researcher and scholar within medical education. This is my location, my experience and my subject position. My account of standardized patients and their professionalizing project is based in lived experience which is at the heart of human simulation. However my telling is also about how different discourses or ideas within medical education have constituted SPs as a fertile site of knowledge production. Possible subject positions for SPs, such as teachers, administrators, and scholars are tied to hierarchies of knowledge that honour scientific certainty and objectivity over subjectivity and non clinical and non scientific perspectives. These hierarchies support and limit their social relations and positions of authority within the field. Historically SPs and SP educators are women, most of whom are not clinicians working within a predominantly masculine, biomedical, scientific paradigm of knowledge production. These elements work together to position SPs as outsiders to medicine in ways that are both productive and constraining. They are "subjects of" and "subjected to" prevailing ideas about medical competence and professionalism In other words SPs are constituted as particular objects within a larger medical education enterprise, (assessment instruments, physical models) and have negotiated strategically from this location a valued place from which to contribute to medical professional socialization processes and clinical knowledge production. I am one such subject whose standpoint as an SP, SP scholar, educator, researcher and administrator, is informed by a particular gendered and racially privileged lens. From this location I am also both "a creator of knowledge and someone who has participated in the construction of history, a person whose life can provide a 'grounding of knowledge claims" (Harding, 1991, p. 47).

1.3 The Problem Space

The problem field within which I am working is embodied, affective, and a site of ethical considerations and practice. The following sections of my thesis outline the key elements of the field of inquiry which include the work of SPs as teachers, their embodied engagement and ethical practice, and emotion and affect as a vehicle that gets used to produce and reproduce normative conceptions of what it means to be a "good doctor". These are the ideas which will be taken up and theorized more fully in the main body of my thesis.

There are many names and definitions for the work in which lay people enact roles for the purposes of teaching and assessment of clinical skills. "Simulated patients, programmed patients, prepared patients, trained patients, standard patients, standardized patients, actors, pseudo patients, patient instructors" (Barrows, 1993). A simulated patient encounter includes any clinical encounter conducted for purely educational purposes that may or may not utilize the simulator's personal medical history. The standardization referred to in the term standardized patient relates to the consistent presentation of verbal and behavioural responses by the SP to stimulus provided by a student or examinee. "A standardized patient encounter is always a simulation but a simulated patient encounter is not necessarily standardized" (Adamo, 2003, p. 262). Shifting power relations are indicated in the trajectory through the various namings.[2]

But again for the sake of clarification, what is a standardized patient? SPs are primarily non-clinicians or lay persons who are engaged extensively within medical education to help teach and assess a range of clinical skills. This being said, one is immediately confounded in trying to understand what standardized patients actually do within the clinical domain of medicine.

1.3.1 Teaching Emotion as Communication Skill

My first engagement as a standardized patient in 1983 (at that time we were called simulated patients) was to portray a dying patient for a second year medical student who was identified as struggling with "delivering bad news". My presence in this teaching site was premised on the idea that compassion was not only an innate internal trait but was teachable. "It was a commonly held belief at this time that communication skills could not be taught but were natural talents – inborn attributes of the 'good doctor' – and a young doctor was endowed with them or not" (Buckman, 2002, p. 672). Buckman states that "mounting evidence has shown clearly that techniques to bring awkward communicators to a reasonable or at least average level are achievable and that these skills can be taught, do change patient satisfaction, and can be retained over time" (p. 672). The logic, which aligns with a cognitive behavioural understanding of emotion best represented by an emotional intelligence framework, holds that if a medical student has enough exposure and practice with both the troubling emotions of the (simulated) patient and his own then the student's emotional competence will improve and be visible through effective communication. This was the main selling point of SP teaching work in those early days – practical skill or "know how" could be improved through experiential practice. It still is a main argument for the value of "human simulation" however there is no longer the resistance that existed in the early 80's to the idea that empathy, rapport, compassion – "the soft skills" – were not only part of an internal fixed personality trait, but could be taught.

My engagement as a tearful and distraught patient in practice with the student reproduced an understanding of emotion as amenable to management techniques performed to achieve appropriate professional behaviour. Another dominant idea, within medical education is, as described above, that "communication skills" are intuitive - the external marker of an internal disposition. This idea is most visible in a medical professionalism literature that focuses on "professional formation" (Rabow, 2010, p. 310) or "character modification", and is tied to the argument that certain abilities are naturally occurring innate indicators of temperament and personality.

The idea that emotion is both a mutable skill and that it is a naturally occurring internal trait perpetuates the use of simulated patients as teachers. Also both of these views frame their main arguments in the medical professionalism literature (Stern, 2006; Klamen & Williams, 2006; Coulehan, 2006; Kao, 2006) serving to perpetuate the idea that emotions are a "problem to be fixed" either through skills training and practice or character reformation. I return to these two main themes in my chapter on emotion and affect. For now I conclude that my participation in this teaching situation also points to an implicit political arrangement between SP and doctor which is authorized in part by discourses related to medicine's notions of skills acquisition and patient centered care.

As mentioned above, standardized patients function as an integral "technology" for teaching and assessment of communication skills. Constituting emotion as a communication skill is the rationale that makes it possible for lay individuals mostly actors, and other artists to participate in medical education and medicine's professionalizing mandates. As proxies for the "real thing", SPs are used as tools by the profession, effectively reproducing prevailing professional ideas about appropriate uses of emotion by both physician and patient. As a corollary of their unique location – neither clinician nor patient, but perpetually a possible patient - they also have privileged access to the emotionally ambiguous world of medical trainee professional socialization.

This location is double edged offering possibilities for legitimation within medical education as "SP educators" through alignments that support dominant professional values as well as opportunities for resistance within the actual emotional and affective labour SPs carry out as lay people. Such antagonism is generative and irreducible to a rational order of exchange and power. In other words, because SPs exist outside of the official clinical realm they are in a position to subvert dominant notions about emotional expectations within their interactions with medical trainees and practicing professionals. For example, through the practice of "teaching in role", which entails responding genuinely in the moment to a student's behaviour, both verbally and non-verbally, SPs are able to create learning that cannot be disciplined or explained through a clinical episteme. I argue that the subversion occasioned by this form of embodied teaching disrupts taken for granted medical professional ideas and practices that have traditionally subordinated patient perspectives and experience.

1.3.2 It begins with a body, my body

> The claim that the body is disavowed in the production of knowledges has implications not only for epistemologists but also for feminist theorists especially for those attempting to criticize and transform traditional patriarchal forms that knowledge has taken so far (Grosz, 1993, p. 187).

My story begins with a body, my body, Rose McWilliams' body, and, as a technology for teaching medical students about the multiplicities of patient experiences - mostly women's bodies. It not only begins with a body but is also principally and in the end, the work of bodies. In the early 1960's Rose McWilliams, an artist's model, took a part time job for a doctor to help in teaching students' about physical examination technique, specifically neurological examination. She was the first documented SP. A certain comfort with her body would have been a prerequisite for the vagaries of students' tentative practice of palpation, percussion and auscultation. Familiarity with anatomy and a willingness to take part in an "indoctrination" (Barrows, 1964, p. 803) process or training program would also have been required. It was her willing presence as a physical model for medical students' practice much as she was for art students that sparked a pedagogical revolution in medical student teaching.

My own involvement as a SP began as a way to make a little extra money. I worked as an actor and dancer and took on many temporary jobs to make ends meet from waitressing/bartending and cleaning houses to teaching stage fighting – all embodied labour. Someone in an acting class told me about an opportunity to make some extra money while getting acting practice and so I applied to the then nascent University of Toronto

Standardized Patient Program. This route through the arts and service industries is still a most common one for a large contingent of SPs. At the beginning I only worked a couple of hours every other week or so totalling about six weeks of work over the course of a year. I took part in all kinds of teaching sessions within medicine involving physical examinations of various sorts, communication skills, and psychiatry counselling sessions. Comfort with my body, a sense of agency, insight into my own experiences, ability to communicate about what I had experienced in role, and a willingness to learn were prerequisites for my continuing involvement. Feedback or the ability to transform my experience into helpful constructive bites of information was central to the teaching and is still the aspect of the work most highly valued. It requires an ability to reflect on an experience as it is happening and to share that information with an interlocutor. Feedback is continuously adaptive and as a practice is also a key site for reproducing normalized conceptions about both patient and doctor roles.

1.3.3 Gendering of a field

Together, acting, women and medicine form a matrix that informs the shape and possibilities for SP work. There was little to suggest the explosive growth that would take place in the simulation field in the 1980's. Populated by mostly women or retirees (white and middle class) with some time on their hands, the standardized patient methodology was shaped predominantly by medical men.

Many of the women who are now considered founders in the field were introduced to it as a unique but peripheral part of their professional work, such as teaching within nursing or social work. Many continued to pursue the work for the same reasons I did; it provided a rich and open ground for learning and creative possibilities. Live simulation did not constitute a profession and was not appealing to anyone looking for a five year plan towards a stable position. In other words it was not seen as an attractive pursuit for most men seeking a legitimate career in medical education, with the exception of a few physician educators who were assisted by women SPs in making their mark in performance assessment research. However, the field of live simulation has since grown and is presently engaged as a dynamic pedagogical, research and assessment methodology in over eighteen countries with over a thousand full time educators and administrators represented by an international Association for Standardized Patient Educators (ASPE). The gender balance has changed with more men plotting career trajectories in medical education through this now established and recognized field and taking up positions of administrative and educational authority within medical schools.

Between 1960 and the1980's medical education as a field was developing innovative methods for scientifically justifiable and reliable educational pathways while struggling for legitimacy and recognition. Howard Barrows', the neurologist credited with inventing simulated patients in 1963 (Wallace, 1997, p 6) saw a role for actors in medical student evaluation and clinical skills practice. The early definition of a simulated/standardized patient with which this chapter opens is one of many that discursively constitute simulated/standardized patients and by extension patients as certain kinds of objects. The body is seen as pliant and if not exactly passive at least obedient. The bodies involved in Howard Barrow's innovation were initially described by the popular press in an article entitled, *Models Who Imitate Patients: Paradise for Medical Students* in sexually tinged language as "scantily clad models [who] are making life a little more interesting for the USC medical students." (cited in Wallace, 1997, p. 6). SP bodies were construed as specifically sexed carrying an illicit aura with them into medical education. Such allusions to promiscuity along with the proximity of SPs to a traditionally questionable world of entertainment threatened the authority and social privilege of the medical profession.

Sexualization of women's bodies as entertainers and models echoes and references the common practice of engaging prostitutes for teaching gynaecological skills to medical students until the mid 60's when they were found to be too expensive (Godkins, 1974, p. 1175). Although not explicitly stated, constructing the service of female non clinician teachers as tools and instruments of learning along sexual lines supports a gendered professional notion of male doctor and female patient. Availability of female bodies for hire coupled with the moral turpitude historically assigned to actresses (Clarke, 1993; Davis, 1991)[3] intersects in an invisible yet powerful sexed construction of a simulated (not yet standardized) patient. Barrows met with a lot of resistance to his new "tool" and was "seen as doing something detrimental to medical education, maligning its dignity with 'actors'" (Wallace, 1997, p. 6). That he persisted is described as a personal virtue however the technology itself produced possibilities that extended beyond Barrows as an individual and changed medical education as a field.

Barrows' starting point was a very specific need for which he created the case of Patty Dugger a paraplegic woman with multiple sclerosis (based on a Los Angeles County hospital patient) (Wallace, 1997, p. 8). He and his colleagues needed to evaluate medical student clinical performance and so Rose McWilliams' first role required training in the portrayal of physical symptoms and signs. Barrow's states "The simulated patient [...] can be exactly the clinical problem the teacher wants. He can be examined serially by a number of students and present exactly the same picture and the same difficulties to every student" (Barrows, 1971, p. 11). Barrows' encounters were designed so that the SPs not only enacted the roles with all of the neurological symptomotology but assessed students' performances according to a pre-determined checklist. As he suggests; "One of the greatest advantages of simulated patients in medicine is their ability to accurately and objectively test clinical performances" (Barrows, 1971, p. 10). An assemblage of technologies was effectively put in place by Barrows including: simulated patient role creation, techniques for training roles, standardizing roles, enacting roles, experiential pedagogical methods, and assessment tools such as checklists and observation protocols, all of which placed SPs at the centre.

Many protocols have been created over the years, legitimizing the educational engagement of human simulation within medical education and effectively distancing the exotic and gendered sensual dimensions that may possibly leak into medical science through interaction with live bodies. The transformation of "simulated" into "standardized" patients is one example. However there remains an active and productive resistance within SP culture at the ground level to being generalized and constructed by medical gaze as a "clinical" object for live demonstration. One way in which this manifests informally or below the threshold of official sanction is in choices SPs make about how and when they respond in role.

As a simulated patient who later became a 'standardized' patient my body like Rose McWilliams' is mediated through a medical gaze and comes to be part of a medical technology through my participation in the aforementioned assemblage. It is often not for the uniqueness of our bodies or our experiences that SPs are valued but for the generalizability of findings that we represent. We embody both a specific patient experience, like that of Patty Dugger, as well as the physiological details of a universalized condition. Subjectification occurs in subtle and not so subtle ways through role constructions and training protocols that reduce patient cases and their standardized portrayals according to psychometric formulations. The role is seen to "perform" quantitatively within a statistical realm just as the SPs "perform" in a corporeal one. It is as if the lives of the patients that SPs enact are a palimpsest, a faint reminder overwritten by the powerful others who shape our work.

However, the materiality of specific bodies is resistant to shaping according to principles of scientific certainty and objectivity. Always fluid - stretching, reacting and forming new connections which are embodied and affective - learning pushes against the idea that procedures of standardization and psychometric calculation can produce a definitive and verifiable knowledge. Both Rose McWilliams' involvement and my own, fifteen years later may be viewed as local events in medical education's professional socialization project.

SPs engage in performance as a form of ethics. As teachers in embodied and affective one-to-one encounters with students, SPs are in a privileged position of being able to create momentary spaces in which learning unique to a particular configuration of student/patient/standardized patient relationship occurs. These moments don't always transpire and cannot be prescribed or sanctioned within the official space within which SPs are acting as the projected ideal of the "medical gaze". However, this is nomadic space that is productive of new understanding. Small moments provide paths to be followed in relationship with the "other's" movements. It is a dance, not a march. As such value resides in different kinds of movement between and within the space of interactions, a topic that will be further explored throughout my thesis.

1.3.4 Teaching Story: Ethics Part I

I am visiting the clinic to meet with a family doctor whom I have never met before to get the results of a breast biopsy. I have been trained to portray a woman who is to be told that she has advanced breast cancer. The student is a family practice resident. We are in a small clinic room being observed through a one way mirror by a staff supervisor. The resident trainee knows that we are being observed and I know that we are being observed but the resident does not know that I know. In other words this is an undercover simulation and I am a real patient to this learner. I don't remember much of what was said during the actual encounter although as a new SP I am sure I am nervous and attempting to remember elements of the interview so that I might provide feedback to the learner. I do remember that the whole event felt very slow and hesitant. The resident was quiet and could barely look at me. I felt like crying but as I remember it I can't figure out if it was out of sadness as an SP about my situation as the patient or whether it was my response to the resident's obvious sadness. As happens in most teaching sessions, feedback is offered following the interview by both the SP and the observing faculty

In hindsight the resident very graciously accepted my observations at the time however she later complained about the deception she experienced. I found out following the session that she had recently in her own life experienced the death of a close family member to breast cancer and suffered a profound sadness over the plight of the patient I was performing. To my knowledge it was the last time such a subterfuge was performed in Toronto and strict ethics protocols for activities involving undercover SP visits have been generally accepted practice within the field for many years now. Why I tell this story is to point out the essentially affective, emotional and relational ethics of the work in which physicians and learners engage and the deep investment such engagements with simulated patients engender.

The possibility of this deceptive educational encounter taking place is based in part on assumptions about authenticity and the nature of reality in simulation that continue as tensions today. The betrayal the resident felt was more than the discomfort that accompanies the acquisition of new knowledge or skills. She was emotionally invested in the interaction and the consequences of her words on me as the patient. I came to realize as I continued working as an SP that it is the emotional, affective and embodied aspects of our engagement with learners' that provide the most significant ethical learning.

How would the encounter have changed if she had known that I was not the "real" patient? The question speaks to ideas about a relationship between authenticity of emotional and affective engagement and the performance of professional behaviours, values and attitudes. It is tricky emotional terrain in which boundaries between "real" and "fake" blur. Both the resident and I were present and experiencing real thoughts and emotions in the setting. As an SP I inhabit physically and emotionally every story I enact, just as a physician is really experiencing their engagement in the story. So although the circumstances are not my own I am the medium through which the story emerges. It is my body that cries and receives the bad news often more than once depending on the assignment. It is a performance and we are both acting our parts. The effects on each of us will be different and of unequal consequence depending on the experiences we bring to the situation. In this situation the resident had every right to feel used by her supervisors and by me for deceiving her as a part of her learning. Emotions can be and are abused in learning situations where they are engaged as tools for humiliation or ignored or reduced to an afterthought. However, as Boler (1999) attests they are an "ever present absence" in much of education; invisible within rationalist objective discourses yet always present.

Emotion is also a factor in assessment activities where standardization rules and measurement dominates. However, the ways in which patient emotions are presented and regulated for assessment exercises are different. Premised on psychometric formulations and the possibility of getting a valid snap shot of an individual's skills from a brief interaction between student and SP, OSCEs –objective structured clinical exams, represent a different normalizing technology than is found within formative settings. Ethics is framed much more explicitly as a demonstration of particular observable skills according to professionalizing norms.

1.3.4.1　　Ethics of representation: Perpetually Possible Patient

How real is real enough? There is an idea that medical professionals only "go through the motions" in an encounter with standardized patients and that this is all that is needed in order to practice the steps, or acquire the skills. If, in the above situation, the resident had known that I was acting, reasoning suggests, she would only go through the movements of acting herself and would not have conducted herself with the same level of compassion and empathy. The accompanying idea is that one needs to be "tricked" into demonstrating authentic behaviour. We were both of us acting and not acting; present within specific roles that subjected us to normalizing ideas about "good doctors" and "good patients." There is a productive paradox in practicing emotions in order to gain control over them while at the same time trying not to actually experience any real emotion for fear of losing professional detachment. This is comparable in part to acting in which the "third eye" or meta cognitive engagement with the role and the acting scene is required. Whether a physician or medical student is "really" taking on a professional role different from their personal life is fertile ground for exploration with educational implications. At this juncture it can be said that all of us negotiate and act many selves throughout a day. It is not a question of authenticity but of the choices we make with respect to the kind of presence we decide to enact. Rather than think in terms of "true states of being", as MargritShildrick (2002) suggests, "the gaze whether of science or entertainment plays a prominent role in discursively constructing all bodies and selves" (p. 24). Training with simulated patients in medical education offers opportunities to explore different choices but also operates as a site of regulation with respect to producing "appropriate" professional demeanour. What was real between the resident and me was our relationship in this one encounter and the immanent movement of the exchange between us. I am a "perpetually possible patient" because I am not a blank slate or raw material to be inscribed anew with each role but bring my many selves and experiences and possible future experiences to the work. The same possibility is true for anyone with whom I interact in role.

Was the resident expected to learn about how to manage her own personal feelings in such a way that they did not interfere with her professional role? As Wear (1997) suggests, "Doctors *control* interviews, procedures, practices. Of course the doctor's body may touch or exhibit other caring gestures, facial expressions or tender tones, but it is a body *in* control of itself" (Wear, 1997, p. 106). SPs contribute to this message by virtue of our presence as representatives of the medical profession but more importantly through the kinds of feedback we are coached to provide about our experiences "in role". SPs gain membership into the medical education club through this work as we align our responses to expectations both clinical and educational about how an encounter "should" proceed and what "should " be produced by way of counselling, management, diagnosis or prescription etc. Medical education gains a pliable and dynamic instrument to disseminate messages about professional values, attitudes and skills. What can be lost as SPs become experts in the "right' clinical findings and the "appropriate" pathways to discover them, are the unpredictable moments, unique within any relationship no matter how fleeting, as SPs constrain their portrayals and toe the medical education line regarding possible authentic behaviours and accompanying emotions. The various subjectivities and power relations authorized by the ideas that support the "use" of individuals in live simulation teaching are complex.

Implicated in this complexity are unspoken ideas and emotional rules that shape the work in which SP educators engage.

1.4 Conclusion

As an embodied emotional and affective presence literally in front of and often in physical contact with medical students and practicing professionals SPs are a site of knowledge production and transformative learning, the effects of which are not always immediately apparent or measureable. As a corollary of both their location as non-clinicians and their pedagogical facility with emotions and affect SPs are integral to the production and reproduction of collective attitudes, values, and beliefs about what it means to be a "good" doctor. Engaging human simulation in medical education involves a practical ethics which is complex with physical, social and political implications for all parties.

1.5. Organization of Thesis

My thesis is organized as follows: In the second chapter I will outline my theoretical influences and sources providing the reader with a sense of the style of the thesis and the lens through which my analysis in the rest of the thesis can be read. Taking Deleuze and Guattari's (1987) "pragmatics" as a main method of analysis I am hoping to evoke feelings as well as thoughts with respect to the ideas put forward. The writings of post structural feminists on emotion as well as Michel Foucault are also essential to my understanding of the movement and ambiguity inherent in the work of standardized patient teachers.

Chapter three provides a close examination of emotion and affect and the work of SPs in medical education. Dominant ideas about emotion and their effects on SPs and medical education are discussed as are ideas about affect and their implications for an embodied praxis.

Chapter four provides a genealogy of medical simulation locating SPs and their role within this larger educational field. A technological imaginary that locates SPs as one of a number of medical simulation modalities as well as the absence/presence of emotion and affect within the field will be examined.

Chapter five presents an alternative mapping of the SP professionalizing project foregrounding its aesthetic alignments with theatre, and medical performances of different kinds. Taking Deleuze and Guattari's cartographic approach I map connections between emotion, affect, simulation acting and medicine with the intent of examining the aesthetic as well as the political implications of SP work.

In chapter six I continue my rhizomatic mapping of SPs' location within medical education employing Deleuze and Guattari's treatise on nomadology as a framework. Deleuze and Guattari's theory of "nomad/war machines" offers me a conceptual language with which to unpack and repack the various forces and relations shaping SP work. Creative possibilities fundamentally unaddressed in any literature on SPs from inside or outside the field are introduced.

In chapter seven I theorize a particular performance of nomadology in which affect and emotion are central media. Through an interactive process of subjecting participants as medical students, my colleague and I created a performance/simulation event in which participants had the opportunity to experience the "medical education" gaze. The effect of privileged perspectives inherent in a western medical practice and scientific method and how these intersected with conceptions of illness/disease states are theorized.

I conclude my thesis in chapter eight with reflections on the implications of my research and my possible contributions to scholarship both in the field of human simulation and medical education.

I will intentionally be taking you the reader "into the weeds" with me in different sections. I am describing here the discomfort of wet feet while being surrounded by tall reeds with no clear vantage point. My path, although it may not be immediately apparent, is an invitation for you to feel as well as think about the work of SPs who teach. Hopefully as I follow intersecting lines of practice and thought there will also be sun and clear skies. My thesis is a non linear reading of influences and effects of ideas, and practices on shaping a unique educational field from within it.

Notes

1. Desiring machines is a term used by Deleuze and Guattari to denote desire as a productive force which creates real change. See page 46 for a fuller description.

2. For an excellent socio cultural history of standardized patients, please see Hodges B., 2005, *The Objective Structured Clinical Examination: A Socio History.* For a history of the standardized patient methodology, Peggy Wallace, (1997). Following the Threads of an Innovation,.*Caduceus.*p. 5 – 28.

3. Tracy Davis's book *Actresses as Working Women: Their Social Identity in Victorian Culture* offers a social history of women's employment in Victorian theatre. See chapter four "the Social Dynamic and 'Respectability'", p. 69-105. Also Norma Clarke's thematic review entitled *from Playthings to Professionals:* the *English Actress from 1660 – 1990* offers insight into the sexualization of women working in theatre.

Chapter 2: Theoretical Influences

2.0   Introduction

This chapter describes the theoretical influences which I engage in my examination of emotion and affect as central media in the work of SPs and the field of simulation more broadly. I will outline the contributions to my thinking made by feminist poststructuralist writers, as well as by Michel Foucault and Gilles Deleuze and Felix Guattari, all of which will be further elaborated in the following chapters. I open the chapter with a story to elucidate some of the key elements of my theoretical approach. The intent of this chapter is to introduce central theoretical concepts and to provide a situated perspective from which the rest of the thesis may be read.

2.1   Affective Mannequin

I sit in a chair opposite a second year medical student who looks terrified. I am waiting for information to be delivered; information I have asked for and which the student is afraid to give me. "I have been in the hospital now for three days and have had a million tests and no one is telling me what is going on." It is supposed to be eleven p.m. and I have called the student (doctor) in to give me some pain medication because my back hurts but in fact I want to talk to someone. "What is going on?" "Have you seen my chart?" I am 35 years old; a mother of two small children with a dependent and indecisive husband. I had breast cancer five years ago but everything was taken out in surgery and I am clear. The student is sitting facing me and is looking down at information on a piece of paper (my chart). When she asks me about my history of breast cancer I say, "My doctor on my last check up said I was clear." After much hesitation, and because she has to, because this is "breaking bad news" day and it is her turn to perform in class observed by her peers and clinician teacher, she tells me that the breast cancer has returned and has metastasized to my spine. In my SP role I have already been told this six times today by six different students. After receiving this devastating news — a pause, a silence, a rupture in the space between us. A lightening flash. I break into laughter, hysterical laughter. I can't catch my breath I am laughing so hard, much to the shocked silence of the student. The "expressive momentum carries a charge of potential too great to be absorbed in any particular thing or event: too much to be born(e). It is for this reason that it has to take body...What absorbs the excess of potential is the determinate functioning of the host body" (Massumi, 2002a, p. xxxii). It is not something I expected or planned for. There is nothing right or wrong about my response as a person inside another's story. It is simply what happens. Without intention or plan I veer into sobbing uncontrollably. The student, still stunned, is now faced with her worst fear – a crying patient. I can see that she is struggling to say something and then realize that in fact she is afraid to in case she starts crying herself – which in fact happens. There is nothing to say. "The force of expression" has struck my body first directly and unmediated. It has passed transformatively through flesh before it becomes instantiated in subject-positions" (Massumi, 2002a, p. xvii), doctor/ patient, role playing student/role playing actor, to be subsumed by a system of power.

There is much to be learned for both of us in this exchange. In what capacity am I present as the body experiencing this event in between us, actor/patient, student /actor? The ambiguity between the role and the real is intentional in this telling. There is a constant tension for me as the person embodying such a story just as there is for the student. "Before the flash there is only potential in a continuum of intensity; a field charged with particles" (Massumi, 2002a, p. xxiv). The exchange is a lightening strike. It doesn't resemble, represent, or reproduce the charged field between us. It culminates it, in a playing out or performing of its intensity. "The doing of the did says it all. It is its everything" (Massumi, 2002a, p. xxv).

Following the scenario there is an unpacking of the affective moment - the tangible and very "unclinical" moment that has passed between us. What happened? The vocabulary to describe what has passed between us does not exist in medical education terminology. It is a singular event belonging to its own conditions of anomaly. It presents an accident in an unusual response, a variation not exhibited by other occurrences with which a propositional system might be tempted to group it according to its resemblances. It is an atypical expression. The movement of expression is itself subjective in the sense that it is self-moving and has determinate effects (Massumi, 2002a. p. xxiv). By this I mean that it is particular and singular in both its expressions and its effects on those involved.

There are no subjects here until they are introduced by the words and terminology related to feedback - "patient centered interviewing" and "communication skills," "Patient" "doctor" "standardized patient" and "student". The affective intensity, its veering labile nature, its speed and uncertainty between our two bodies is an event [...]" (Deleuze & Guattari, 1987, p. 262). To teach around this experience is a fragile endeavour. The student may feel betrayed as she rationalizes that she is not supposed to feel anything for a fake patient who is not really in the circumstances that she portrays and is "just acting". And yet the student does feel something. Her body is implicated in this exchange in ways that she will carry away with her for the rest of the day or week, as is mine. We are both engaged in an exchange that has cut through layers of what we consider our stable "selves". A personal line has been crossed and I the standardized patient am the betrayer. We are desiring subjects on a plane of immanence[1] she and I, populating it with affects and intensities, histories and expectations. "In a Deleuzian metaphysics desire is present in all interactions and intersections and is productive – a social force" (Boler, 1996, p. 4). We are both embodiments of suddenly captured emotion. This is more than an objective scientific undertaking.

In human simulation, emotion and affect are embodied media through which learning is experienced. Affect is engaged pedagogically both during an interaction and afterward, facilitating understanding and experience of emotion within specific socio-political relations. They are central to the work of enacting patient stories and in teaching about the social, cultural and political effects of illness at the intersection of medicine and a patient's lived reality. In this context emotion is very much a medium through which particular ideas about what it means to be a "good doctor" become internalized as common sense truth(s) (Boler 1999). This kind of human interaction as a core pedagogical vehicle crosses boundaries both personal and professional. As an embodied enactment that is contingent, multiple and shifting it constitutes emotion and affect as collaborative terrain that has political as well as social implications.

2.2   Theorizing Emotion and Affect

I argue that within the profession of medicine emotion sits uneasily at the intersection between objective scientific fact and subjective humanistic values, while affect is framed primarily as a diagnostic descriptor. Within medical education emotion is widely acknowledged as a core element of professional values, attitudes and beliefs and humanistic approaches to professional activities – counselling, patient management, and communication. It is also recognized as an essential aspect of professional well-being and patient satisfaction. However, ideas about emotion are largely taken for granted or superficially theorized with respect to the social and cultural dimensions with few proponents venturing beyond individualized psychological models. These ideas have material implications.

Likewise affect, understood largely as a physical marker of pathology, limits the possibilities for learning from a growing field of scholarship within the humanities and social sciences. Clough (2007) goes so far as to suggest we are experiencing an "affective turn" which she identifies as a play on the other "turns" that have taken place in recent decades: the "linguistic turn", the "cultural turn" and so forth (Clough, 2007, p. ix). This implies the importance of affect as a cultural and political force and no longer only a descriptor of human experience. I contend that the growing body of theory that incorporates ideas about affect as a socio-political force as well as embodied practice is valuable for expanding and enriching our understanding about the place of affect in discussions of human simulation as a pedagogical practice embedded in medical education.

Emotion is a taken for granted object of both specialized knowledge and everyday discourse (Lutz & Abu-Lughod, 1990). As an object of study it is notoriously difficult to delineate with little agreement between professions, disciplines or fields about what it is, where it resides, how it works and what its effects may be. For example, it is variously described as physiologically determined, (Darwin, 1872; Damasio, 1994; LeDoux,

1996), internal and natural, (Gardner, 1985; Goleman, 1995), a cognitive component of reason, (Descartes, 1650; Lazarus, 1991; Spencer, 1862), essential to moral reasoning and agency, (Aristotle, 1970/350 BCE; Hume, 1711; Spinoza, 1632), a medium for the transmission of socio cultural values and/or the result of socio-cultural practices (Boler, 1999; Hall 1997; Hochschild, 1983; Kemper, 1993; Lutz, &Luhgod, 1990; Zembylas, 2005), a performance, (Bhaba, 1987;Butler, 2005; Foucault, 1980) or central to aesthetic and moral experience, (Greene, 1973; Noddings 1984; Nussbaum, 1996). This is not meant as an exhaustive list but rather to provide a sense of the great interest in emotion across disciplines, professions, and fields over thousands of years. Each of the many views constructs emotion and affect in ways that make particular actions and roles possible while constraining others.

2.3. Theoretical Influences

2.3.1 Feminist Post structuralism

> The connections that have assembled teachers into being who they are perceived to be, owe something to emotion discourses, pedagogical practices, professional codes and power relations in teaching (Zembylas, 2005, p. 213).

According to Michalinos Zembylas (2005) in *Teaching with Emotion: A Postmodern Enactment,* what is "missing [in theorizing of teacher emotion], is attention to political and cultural issues..." He continues, "Feminist theorists along with others... show us how emotions are not constructed from nothing but are controlled, shaped and challenged in particular ways for particular purposes" (p.16).

Studying emotion in medical education through a critical poststructuralist lens specifically influenced by the writing of critical feminists, (Ahmed, 2004; Grosz, 1993; Boler, 1999; Braidotti, 2004; Wear, 1997; Jagger, 1989) means that I am interested not only in what "emotion is" as an object of study or what "emotions and affect are" as phenomena but also in how they are theorized as embodied and political forces. How do various concepts of emotion get used to produce and reproduce practices, objects, concepts, rules and positions of authority? According to Catherine Lutz an anthropologist who studies emotion, "Concepts of emotion serve ideological functions, that is, they exist within a system of power relations which the concept's use has played a part in maintaining" (Lutz, 2007, p. 20). What this implies is that emotion as a category is constituted in specific ways by different groups for particular theoretical but also professional reasons with political consequences. The question that emerges is what ideas about emotion count as truth and who gets to decide? How do such ideas shape affective possibilities for both SP and health professional?

Power, culture and ideology are central to feminist poststructuralist approaches to analyzing emotion and affect.

> Power operates visibly and invisibly through expectations and desires. It operates visibly through public criteria that must be satisfied. It operates invisibly through the way individuals think of themselves and act, as it helps to shape subjective feelings and beliefs. As a result we are objects of social institutions and processes while we intentionally engage in meaningful behaviour" (Cherryholmes, 1988, p. 36).

Subjectification here refers to the complex ways in which humans are constituted within historically and culturally specific sites where power, truth and knowledge are interrelated (Tamboukou, 2002).

Such an approach attempts to avoid talking about hard and fast truths instead theorizing from a socially situated point of view that emotion is not private or universal, but constituted through how we speak and come to know the world. Power relations are relevant to emotion and its expression in clinical training and the ways in which it is authorized or evacuated as Boler suggests; "Power relations are inherent in emotion talk and shape the expression of emotions by permitting us to feel some emotions while prohibiting others" (Zembylas, 2005, p. xii).

An important aspect of the work of poststructuralist feminist theories is to scrutinize binary oppositions in order to get at what has been erased, silenced and rejected in the non-knowledge of the second term of any dualism (Orner, 1992, p. 78). Orner suggests that,

> Dualisms which we contend with daily and which ignore the complexity and interrelatedness of the terms exemplify a mode of thought which essentializes and constructs as opposites, terms that are used to naturalize power relations. Binary oppositions such as ....man/woman, sense/nonsense, reason/madness, rational/irrational are inadequate and dangerous as they oversimplify the meaning behind the terms and relation between them, always set up in such a way as to privilege the first term over the second (Orner, 1992, p.78).

This work challenges the notion that emotions, feelings and bodies are in opposition to cognition, rationality and the mind. Feminist theories question the political motivation behind such dichotomies and the hierarchical control they imply. Cartesian dualities are central to a dominant western viewpoint and are perpetuated in part by the effects of scientific and technological developments that find "emotion as a corruption of reason that needs to be transcended" (Williams, 2001, p. xvi). Williams suggests that reason, on the other hand, is regarded as indispensable for the acquisition of truth. Deconstructing deeply held dualisms situated in dominant discourses in medical education may help reveal taken for granted assumptions about emotion in teaching, the implications of these assumptions for the emotion work of SP teachers and the conditions in which these assumptions are reproduced or disrupted. Deleuze and Guattari's radical praxis enliven this discussion through an alternative ontological reading of difference in which movement inherently produces new relations of possibility.

Critical feminist poststructuralist approaches to the study of pedagogy are committed to supporting multiple viewpoints, the locations of which are situated, contingent and shifting. They honour perspectives that are not recognized as legitimate i.e. rational scientific, objective, provable, reliable, and valid, expressions of knowledge but are rather voices that count not only in the academy but in the world. The perspectives are expansive and inclusive about expressions of knowledge beyond the rationalist to include the emotional. Consistent with this approach in the following chapters I tell my stories, not as confessions, but as an attempt to locate my experiences within a larger social context of medical education and from which I can critically examine the ideas and practices that reproduce hegemonic professional practices. Finally my theoretical approach recognizes that emotions are performed within specific socio-historical contexts related to culture, institutional location and the discourses that define emotional rules and labour.

2.3.2 Foucauldian Contributions

I am not writing a history of standardized patients or standardized patient methodology but rather adopting in part a genealogical approach which is intended to provide a, "history of the present", a "history of events" as disparate, random "material conjunctions of things or processes" (Foucault, 1972, p. 1982). I say *in part* because I am engaging Foucault's ideas in conjunction with others, in ways that make sense to my exploration of emotion, affect and standardized patients as products of specific practices. I am mapping discontinuities in practices with subsequent theorizing, honouring both Foucault's and Deleuze's practice of beginning in the middle or "milieu" in French, with its wonderful sense of not only "the "middle" of something… and something "in the middle" of its operation, but as the medium or environment of its development, "in the midst" of everything else" (Joughin, 1990, note 11, p. 197). I am recognizing the ephemeral nature of knowledge and truth and acknowledging them as contingent and the product of struggles that have taken place. In place of the traditional approach of historian's to search for origins Foucault's genealogy recognizes the partiality that underlies what we come to accept as knowledge. My thesis is informed by examining the professional and institutional forces that have subjected SPs as a particular site of knowledge production.

"What [a genealogy] really does is to entertain the claims of attention of local, discontinuous, disqualified, illegitimate knowledges against the claims of a unitary body of theory which would filter, hierarchize and order them in the name of true knowledge..." (Foucault, 1976, p. 83). Foucault's genealogical approach offers me a way to sift established explanations and taken for granted assumptions that underpin the field of human simulation and SPs as produced through societal and institutional discourses. According to Tamboukou (2008) in her article, *Writing Genealogies; an exploration of Foucault's strategies for doing research,* genealogies don't only focus on the war of discourses and power relations but..."aim to provide a counter-memory that will help subjects recreate the historical and practical conditions of their existence" (p. 203).

My use of the term discourse within this thesis refers to language and ways of speaking but also as Foucault suggests to "practices that systematically form the objects of which they speak" (Foucault, 1972, p 49). Emotion and standardized patients are such objects constituted through both the language that is used to describe them as well as through particular practices. Such a view is a reminder that we are all partial and shifting stories acted upon and acting upon the social fields within which we operate.

Discourses exist co-extensively, at the same time and in the same place, competing for dominance over knowledge claims and influencing who gets to say which knowledge(s) count. They exist within systems of power relations with material implications such as access to resources – equipment, money, positions of authority, as well as unwritten agreements about who gets to speak and who makes the rules. With respect to emotion and affect we see dominant western ideas about their internal and individualized essence informing pedagogical practices and possibilities for SP practitioner interactions. Discourses affect socialization processes and training practices embedded both formally and informally in curricular structures.

Although Foucault never wrote specifically about emotion or affect, in his later work he describes passion in a way that is evocative of Deleuze's idea of haeccaeity[2] "as a sort of process, event or effect of individuation through waves of intensity in continuous variation" (Robinson, 2003, p. 119). His later genealogical exploration of passion as a circulating force parallels Deleuze and Guattari's radical ontology of becoming in its theorizing of being and modes of existing beyond oneself, as a capacity outside of knowledge, identity and truth. However, Foucault's is an epistemological contribution to my thinking as he has helped focus my analysis on how power circulating as a force within medical education effects the work in which SPs acting as teachers engage. Deleuze and Guattari follow a fundamentally different philosophical trajectory from Foucault; one in which they posit a radical ontological reading of Nietzsche and Spinoza. The adaptation of these theorists' ideas by Deleuze and Guattari constructs knowledge as the differing quantities of force tied to living. This force functions as dynamic phenomena constituting a world, driven by desire and our capacity as living beings to affect and be affected. Their formulation is described in more detail below.

2.3.3 Deleuze and Guattari

Deleuze and Guattari's contribution to my thesis is specific to their writing in *a thousand plateaus* (1987)in which they elaborate a vocabulary and conceptual framework that has helped me map out the different dynamics within the work of SPs, their relationship to the larger field of medical education and the institutions to which they are connected. Deleuze and Guattari's radical revisioning of power as desire, and subjectivity as "becomings", has provided me with a compelling perspective through which to map the affective work in which SPs engage as well as to imagine the political and ethical possibilities of future creations.

According to Deleuze and Guattari desire is a productive force that produces reality, and affect is a material manifestation that is irreducible to an individual and circulates as a capacity "to affect and be affected"[3]. Within this understanding the teaching in which SPs engage emerges as a possible form of nomadic ethics; situated and attached to their relationships with each other, to the students with whom they engage and to larger social concerns. An aesthetic as well as a political understanding of SP work and the role of emotion and affect is made possible.

Deleuze and Guattari do not theorize emotion directly but rather speak of affect, emphasizing, "movement", "speeds", "lines of flight", and "machines" that proliferate connections among natural and technical flows. "These relations, movements, orientations and connections among bodies produce new maps of thinking and new life through difference" (Colebrook, 2006:115). I have turned to Deleuze and Guattari's work in *A Thousand Plateaus (1987)* as suggested by Colebrook's quote in order to help me convey the movement and connections across differences that SP teaching entails.

2.3.3.1   Pragmatics: Nomad Thought

Most importantly Deleuze and Guattari provide a way of working with their concepts and vocabulary they call "pragmatics". Pragmatics is a method of engaging with the world that is both generative and transformational, necessitating action and not simply reflection or interpretation. As such it is both method – an application of linkages and movements, and, a set of ideas. It interrupts binaries and representational thinking in order to enable knowledges to be recognized as valuable for their differences and creative potential.

> Nomad thought goes by many names. Spinoza called it "ethics". Nietzsche called it the "gay science". Artaud called it "crowned anarchy"....Foucault called it "outside thought"....Deleuze and Guattari employ the term "pragmatics" and "schizoanalysis" (Massumi, 1987, p. xiii).

Deleuze and Guattari's philosophy is to be "felt" and "acted" as much as "thought". They describe it as a "pragmatics". According to Massumi (1987) the goal of Deleuze and Guattari's pragmatics "is the invention of concepts that do not add up to a system of belief or an architecture of propositions that you either enter or you don't, but instead pack a potential in the way a crowbar in a willing hand envelopes an energy of prying" (p. xv). In this framing, "The concept has no subject or object other than itself. It is an act" (Massumi, 1987, p. xiii). Pragmatics is about the material effects of ideas and actions and what they make possible in the world. A concept then is a brick, "...a vector: the point of application of a force moving through space at a given velocity in a given direction" (Massumi, 1987, p. xiii). This approach helps me as a researcher, artist and teacher who is actively questioning and creating maps and symphonies rather than explaining and interpreting ideas in the abstract and ideological.

Deleuze and Guattari do not begin their philosophical inquiry from the question of what can we know? Or how accurate are the images we have of the world? They do not begin from a mind or consciousness that must somehow come to know or find itself in the world. "Rather life is perception or a power to relate and image" (Colebrook, 2006, p.5). Like Foucault, Deleuze rejects origins and the possibility of beginning with rational "man" to theorize life and difference. However rather than accepting that there are systems and structures of meaning that shape our subjectivities as does Foucault, Deleuze theorizes "sense" as the "surface that allows us access to the imagined world but which we will never be able to experience directly unmediated by culture" (Colebrook, 2006, p.116). Working with concepts such as "sense", "desire", and "difference" introduces the body into Deleuze's philosophy in a way very different from Foucault's later work on care of the self.[4]

2.4 Definitions

Before moving further I would like to clarify some of the terminology that I have begun to use and will be using in the remainder of the thesis. The language Deleuze and Guattari developed in producing their "new maps of thinking" and being can be disorienting. In many cases phrases such as "Bodies without Organs (BwO)" are engaged by Deleuze and Guattari in ways that mean to produce visceral effect as well as conceptual understanding. The obscurity of Deleuze and Guattari's vocabulary "deterritorializes" our understanding with concepts overlapping and relating to each other almost architecturally. In other words they invite readers to abandon mundane attachments to words in order to engage with them in ways that produce new realities. Where possible in my thesis I have outlined concepts as I have used them with accompanying notes however there are terms that act almost as gateways to understanding the strange terrain in which Deleuze and Guattari play which I briefly describe below.

2.4.1 Rhizome

Rhizomes are weed like growths which proliferate between and among things. This is true of plant, animal and conceptual activity.

> The rhizome connects any point to any other point…It is not the multiple derived from the One, nor is it reducible either from the One or the multiple. It is composed not of units but of dimensions or rather directions in motion. It has neither beginning nor end, but always a middle (milieu) from which it grows and which it overspills (1987, p. 21).

In other words it is completely open to entry and exit and multiple connections as a process. This concept is put in relation to "arborescence" as another system of thought which is described as ordered and moving from a central root system in one direction. It is used by Deleuze and Guattari in reference to State thought, (see below) in opposition to nomad thought which is described as rhizomatic. "Rhizomes are not roots, but underground stems. They affirm what is excluded from western thought and reintroduce reality as dynamic, heterogeneous and nondichotomous;

they implicate rather than replicate, they propagate, displace, join, circle back, fold" (O'Riley, 2003, p. 27).

2.4.2 Multiplicity

Of the many principles that comprise rhizomes, the third principle of multiplicity connects to a number of other important concepts "rhizomatically" if you will. "A multiplicity has neither subject nor object, only determinations, and dimensions that cannot increase in number without the multiplicity changing in nature" (Deleuze & Guattari, 1987, p. 8). Multiplicities have to do with the quality of connections made between ideas that are described as intensities, speeds, temperatures, in the non linear pathways that a rhizomatic analysis produces. As well multiplicities proliferate along and produce different lines which can be followed. "There are no points or positions in a rhizome, such as those found in a structure, tree or root. There are only lines" (Deleuze & Guattari, 1987, p. 8).

2.4.3 Lines Molar, Molecular and Lines of Flight

> There are at least three of them: a line of rigid and clear segmentarity; a line of molecular segmentarity; and an abstract line, a line of flight no less deadly and no less alive then the others....The three lines, however continually intermingle (Deleuze & Guattari, 1987, p. 197-198).

Rigid lines of molar segmentarity work through stratifying, organizing, signifying and attributing and align with arborescent models of thought which are linear connecting ideas back to a coherent whole or root. Such lines are represented by reasoning of the "State apparatus" and its "royal science" which rests on normalizing forms that organize matter and thought by means of templates and evidence.

> Not only are the great molar aggregates segmented (States, institutions, classes), but so are people as elements of an aggregate, as are feelings, as relations between people; they are segmented, not in such a way as to disturb or disperse, but on the contrary to ensure and control the identity of each agency, including personal identity […] (Deleuze & Guattari, 1987, p. 195).

Molecular lines are more supple and are "run through and swept up by *micromovements*, fine segmentations distributed in an entirely different way [than a molar segmented line]. "It is on this line that a present is defined whose very form is the form of something that has already happened, however close you might be to it, since the ungraspable matter of that something is entirely molecularized, travelling at speeds beyond the ordinary thresholds of perception. (Deleuze & Guattari, 1987, p. 196). We are in full Deleuze and Guattari speak now. This molecular line "passes between things, between points" (1987, p. 505). Deleuze and Guattari speak about deterritoralization or a moving away from familiar territory that occurs through movement made possible along this line. What is important about the molecular line is that along it learning is experienced as the "making strange" that occurs when entering into relationships with new experiences and knowledge. It is also here and in "lines of flight" that the cultural political aspects of affect are located.

Finally "lines of flight" are creative pathways that can be created or followed. Pure affective energy explodes in multiplicities depending on who is drawing the line or who is caught in it. This line represents a risk related to deterritoralization that offers no return. It is the line of artists, schizophrenics and heroin addicts and is the most dangerous for it produces and thrives on intensities and material effects. "There is nothing imaginary, nothing symbolic about a line of flight. Lines of flight are realities; they are very dangerous for societies…and are immanent to the social field" (1987, p. 203). They are as different as those who invent them and represent both the most creative and the most destructive of forces. "The line of flight of children leaving a school is very different from that of demonstrators being chased by police. There are different animal lines of flight: each species, each individual has its own" (Deleuze & Guattari, 1987, 202). It does not represent a line of escape but may become one. It is integrally interwoven with Deleuze and Guattari's ontological formulation of "becomings" which will be described in a later chapter.

One last aspect to include with respect to the description of lines is the plane of consistency or composition which Deleuze and Guattari refer to as the mode of connection that provides the means of increasing the number of relationships as well as their various becomings, and intensities. "We call this plane, which knows only longitudes and latitudes…..the plane of consistency or composition (as opposed to the plane of organization or development). It is necessarily a plane of immanence and univocality"(Deleuze & Guattari, 187, p. 266). A plane of immanence then is where things happen in the moment.

2.4.4 Haecceity

Haecceity is a concept at the heart of Deleuze's radical ontology of becomings. It refers to a body as defined by a singularity at the level of atoms and molecules that correspond only to movements and affects. "On the plane of consistency, *a body is defined only by a longitude and latitude*: in other words the sum total of material elements belonging to it under given relations of movement and rest, speed and slowness (longitude); the sum total of the intensive affects it is capable of at a given power or degree of potential (latitude)" (1987, p.260). It is entirely relational. "It is a mode of individuation very different from that of a person, subject, thing or substance" (261). He goes on to describe it: "A season, a winter, a summer, an hour, a date have a perfect individuality lacking nothing, even though this individuality is different from that of a thing or a subject. They are haecceities in the sense that they "consist entirely of relations of movement and rest between molecules or particles, capacities to affect and be affected" (1987, p.261). "It is the entire assemblage in its individuated aggregate that is a haecceity; it is this assemblage that is defined by a longitude and latitude, by speeds and affects independently of forms and subjects which belong to another plane(1987, p. 262).

2.4.5 Assemblages

> An assemblage is precisely this increase in the dimensions of a multiplicity that necessarily changes in nature as it expands its connections (Deleuze & Guattari, 1987, p.8).

Assemblages are differentiated by flows and lines. Deleuze and Guattari describe them as constellations of singularities and traits deducted from the flow – selected, organized, stratified – in such a way as to converge (consistency) artificially and naturally; an assemblage in this sense is a veritable invention" (Deleuze & Guattari, 1987, p. 406). "Assemblages are passional, they are compositions of desire…The rationality and efficiency of an assemblage does not exist without the passions the assemblage brings into play, without the desires that constitute it as much as it constitutes them" (Deleuze & Guattari, 1987, p. 399). They create different realities and multiple possibilities.

2.4.6 Desire

Desire for Deleuze and Guattari, like power for Foucault, is fundamentally positive and productive in nature – "one of productive plenitude of its own energy which propels it to seek ever new connections and instantiations and is best theorized as a kind of dynamic machine" (Best &Kellner, 1991, p. 86). In Deleuze's analyses, "desire is regarded as an autonomous and productive force shaping the social rather than being determined by it" (Tamboukou, 2003, p. 218). In fact Deleuze and Guattari insist that desire is a machine that produces things ("alliances" and reality itself) and runs in discontinuous fluxes and "break flows", always making connections with ("partial") objects and other desiring machines (Best &Kellner, 1991, p. 86). As Deleuze and Guattari have written, "If desire produces, its product is real. If desire is productive it can be productive only in the real world and can produce only reality" (Deleuze & Guattari, 1983, p. 26).

The notion of the "desiring machine" works to deconstruct traditional dichotomies between subjective and objective, reality and fantasy. "Seeking inclusive rather than exclusive relations desire is a free flowing physical energy that establishes random fragmented and multiple connections with material flows and partial objects" (Best &Kellner, 1991, p. 86). The affective dimension of power in Foucault "forms rhizomes with the Deleuzian notion of desire and becoming" (Patton, 2000 p. 53, cited in Tamboukou, 2003, p. 218). "As has been suggested, power for

Foucault like desire for Deleuze and Guattari permeates all social relations and penetrates the body" (Tamboukou, 2003, p. 218). However, an important difference between Deleuze, Guattari and Foucault with respect to their perspectives on power and desire is clarified in *a thousand plateaus*.

> Our only points of disagreement with Foucault are the following: (1) to us the assemblages seem fundamentally to be assemblages not of power but of desire (desire is always assembled), and power seems to be a stratified dimension of the assemblage...." (1987, p. 530-31, n. 39).

According to Zembylas (2007) in *Risks and Pleasures: A Deleuzo-Guattarian pedagogy of desire on education;* "The sort of curriculum that would foster the engagement of desire is more likely to have the body at the centre of teaching and learning, enhancing opportunities for emotional and bodily expression" (2007, p. 342). Paradoxically this aspect of teaching and learning in the health professions although necessarily present is instrumentalized and shaped by scientific and objectified discourses. The manner in which a Deleuzian approach addresses relationships between the body and the irrational begin with the experience of relationships and explore what they produce rather than looking at the structures within which they are situated.

2.4.7 Royal Societies/Royal Science

Deleuze and Guattari use these terms in *a thousand plateaus* (1987) to describe official state sanctioned approaches to explaining and solving problems. Royal science stands in direct opposition to nomad science. Deleuze and Guattari state, "What we have, rather, are two formally different conceptions of science, and, ontologically a single field of interaction in which royal science continually appropriates the contents of vague or nomad science while nomad science continually cuts the contents of royal science loose" (Deleuze & Guattari, 1987, p. 367). They continue, "The concern of the man of the State, or one who sides with the State is to maintain a legislative and constituent primacy for royal science" (p. 367). These terms reference the French Académie Royale des Sciences established in France in 1666 as a learned society overseeing impartial scholarly science.

I have introduced these concepts and terms in order to provide some orientation for the experiential nature of the reading that will follow and to describe the various relations of force within the field I am exploring with the intention of helping you negotiate the weeds as I tell my story.

2.5 Affect and Simulation in Medical Education

How are affect, emotion and desire implicated in the specific practices of teaching through live simulation in medical education? The very question needs to be conceptualized in a way that recognizes the transformative and relational nature of affective learning.

> In its encounter with the Nietzschean notion of power as further elaborated by Foucault, the power/desire couplet could perhaps unfold itself as a set of forces suffusing and unsettling pedagogic

> relationships, making trouble for the long held hierarchies of knowledge regimes (Tamboukou, 2003, p. 220).

Desire produces pedagogy as it produces subjects. "A pedagogy of desire is therefore not based on a notion of desire as being a state, position, or feeling towards teaching and learning practices, but it is pedagogy of the subject and the relation between subjects and objects and artifacts" (Zembylas, 2007, p. 338).

In framing an understanding about the affective work in which SP teachers engage from a Deleuzian perspective, desire is part of the ongoing conversation that occurs over time with various "others", rather than affect becoming part of an instrumental and objectified approach to learning as "skills acquisition".

> A pedagogy of desire is not bound to any set of 'best teaching practices' or 'appropriate learning skills. Such a pedagogy neither privileges the individual nor ignores it. Instead of trying to situate them in a dialectic context, a pedagogy of desire aims to explore the various social, aesthetic, material and political manifestations of one's existence and its connection to others (Zembylas, 2007, p. 340).

Such an approach creates a space for discovery and the development of an ethics through aesthetics. "Education has always been constituted as a significant locus of resistance, a smooth space for forces of deterritoralization to be released" (Tamboukou, 2003, p. 220). Thinking differently about emotion and affect in the teaching in which SPs engage can encourage us to follow lines of flight away from stagnant habits and towards collaborative affective inquiry (Boler 1996).

2.6 Conclusion

As I have described in this chapter emotion and affect can be seen as a landscape on which medical professional, practical, moral, and ethical considerations get played out. The work in which simulated/standardized patients engage is pedagogically unique in that emotion and affect is central to the work. As media through which learning is engaged and experienced SPs are required to understand, experience, perform and talk about emotions specific to a clinical and personal situation that is not their own.

I have introduced key ideas of critical feminist poststructuralists, Michel Foucault and Gilles Deleuze and Felix Guattari to which I will be returning in the rest of my thesis. Each of the various theories with which I am working could alone frame my thinking, however the ways in which they accord and bump up against each other is fruitful to my project of opening up different lines of inquiry into the largely under theorized domain of human simulation in education. Further elaboration of the ideas and their intersection with each other and my project will be engaged in the following chapters.

"Poststructuralist thought is not bound to reason, but 'to discourse,' literally narratives of the world that are admittedly partial" (Ellsworth 1989, p. 96). The narratives which I include as part of my examination are also not solely bound by rules of academic rationalism but are shaped by emotionally embedded experiences that are admittedly partial, contextually situated and materially specific. My approach to the study of emotion and affect in medical education acknowledges movement in all its formsas central: institutional, social, political, and personal. Cast always as contingent, immanent, dependent, and forever incomplete, our knowledge and our endeavours are stories to be told not truths to be unearthed. Together these viewpoints support and extend my theoretical understanding of human simulation and its place within medical education in crucial ways.

In the following chapter I examine how different ideas about emotion and affect produce professional socialization processes in medical education and the ethical implications for an embodied educational practice of human simulation.

Notes

1. See definitions section of this chapter for explanation of planes of immanence.

2. Haecceities is a concept at the heart of Deleuze's radical ontology of becomings. It refers to a body as defined by a singularity at the level of atoms and molecules that correspond only to movements and affects. See definitions section this chapter.

3. The idea of the "capacity to affect and be affected" originates in the work of Burach Spinoza and his philosophy of vitalism. See Benedict De Spinoza, (c. 1677). *Ethics*. Edited and Tranlsated by Edwin Curley. London. Penguin Books.

4. 'The care of the self' is one of the final themes in Foucault's work which was left unfinished, however was developed within his wider project of a writing a genealogy of the desiring subject more widely covered as his "History of Sexuality (Foucault 1976, 1986).

Chapter 3 Affect, Emotion, Standardized Patients & Medical Education

3.0   Introduction: Nomadic Ethics

In this chapter I pick up threads and examine more closely how emotion and affect are theorized within medical education and the implications for the different perspectives on the work SPs and the professional socialization processes in which they are engaged.

I examine how different ideas about emotion and affect produce professional socialization processes in medical education. Linking these ideas to human simulation and the activities in which SPs engage, I examine how they may act as a prime vehicle for producing an engaged and embodied praxis. I am separating my examination of emotion from that of affect in the following analysis for organizational purposes, with the understanding that although helpful for the reader to do so, affect and emotion in reality are not easily teased apart and are essentially inter-related along a continuum. "Affects are not only attached to bodies but circulate as capacities... irreducible to the individual, the personal or the psychological" (Clough, 2007, p. 2). Similarly emotion although physiological and psychological is also a socio-cultural medium through which truths get produced and circulated.

My main question in this chapter is: Is it possible to revisit and revalue the emotional and affective dimensions of medicine's socialization processes as a "nomadic ethics?" (Braidotti, 2006, p.4). A nomadic ethics described by Braidotti involves a materialist approach to affectivity and a non-unitary space – "a contested space of mutations that follow no technological directives and no moral imperatives" (2006, 4). "It involves a non-unitary subjectivity that is none the less functional, coherent and accountable mostly because it is embedded and embodied" (2006, p. 4). Such an ethics is premised on processes of becoming and have the possibility of bringing about learning that is inclusive of a broad range of difference.

Nomadic assemblages as understood by Deleuze are "passional" meaning that they produce relationships based on the movement of following rather than forcing according to preconceived truths or notions of right and wrong. Assemblages constructed through hierarchical systems of western scientific understanding teach us that we ought to aim at control *over* things, control over nature, and even control over diseases, and diseased persons. In biomedicine we can imagine nurses and other health professionals in this hierarchy just as we can imagine SPs becoming coded in terms of assemblages of biomedical understandings. A nomadic ethics mobilizes nomadology to create assemblages through an ethics of mutually nourishing relationships rather than subjectifying relationships (Magnusson, 2011, p.158)[1]. For example, emotion and affect are always between individuals and the social as a mediating force with a complex and contingent status as social and political effects

3.1 Emotion and Affect in Medical Education

Although affect and emotion are integrally interwoven into all aspects of the work of SPs they are largely unexamined or superficially theorized concepts within medical education. They are present in their absence, for despite the emotional and affective work involved in all aspects of clinical decision making and day to day interactions, emotion and affect are construed as private territory, internal to the individual and therefore largely invisible. Knowledge of emotion and affect in medical education is contingent on gendered, normative and dichotomized constructions - positive and nurturing vs. negative and destructive. Dichotomies are used productively to maintain boundaries around emotion and its expression as signs of professionalism - moral sensibility and intelligence. Separating emotion off as a separate entity effectively makes a large range of experience invisible and therefore absent from discussion, except in instances of leakage of one sort or another. Also, as Boler (1996) points out, rationality itself "poses as an absence of emotion" despite it being "replete with feeling" (p. 6). Further, disparagement of both emotion and affect as illegitimate forms of knowledge (seen as both gendered and unscientific) in clinical training has led to a paucity of critical thinking and meaningful contributions in the area thereby further diminishing their visibility and viability in educational and professional contexts.

Emotion it can be said then is hidden in plain sight, with few proponents venturing beyond psychological models, while affect remains locked in a diagnostic category attached to pathology. A Western view of emotion that makes it invisible is divorced from the particularities of material consequences and serves a number of functions. It reinforces a gendered notion of emotion and affect that exists within a system of power relations which the concept's use plays a part in maintaining. As I have described it, identifying emotion as primarily irrational, subjective, chaotic and dangerous while in subtle and not so subtle ways identifying women as "emotional" reinforces subjugating ideas and practices related to both emotion and gender (Shildrick, 2002).

Ideas about emotion and affect as they relate to medical professional socialization activate particular assumptions that produce and reproduce professional expectations about emotion and affect in practice. At the same time emotion as normative construct shapes the dimensions and possibilities for learning.

3.2 Emotion in Medical Education

Emotion is at the core of the medical professional ideal. And there is a well documented gap or two, between the norms that support a professional conception of the "good" doctor in Western culture - meaning empathic, caring and until recently male and predominantly white - and the processes by which students are expected to acquire the ideal. (Bryden et al, 2010; Hafferty, 2000; Hafferty and Castellani, 2009; Lewis, 2006; Wear, 1997, 2006). This is evident in the specialized medical language that students are socialized into in order to be recognized as legitimate medical professionals. "Indeed when patients are discussed during grand rounds and other teaching conferences, it is often in terms of laboratory data. And when the story that the patient gives (the subjective soft stuff) conflicts with the lab data (the objective hard stuff), the patient's story is often given less credibility" (Wear, 1997, p. 93). What effect is produced by the idea that to be a "good" doctor one must evacuate emotion from reason or at very least be able to titrate it accordingly for the patient's benefit in the form of "detached concern"? A predominant view of emotion integral to shaping medical professionalism sees emotion as a skill and/or ability which may be used to justify particular decisions and actions.

3.2.1 Emotion: as Interpersonal Technique

> I am sorry my amygdala is completely out of control (Female, 2nd year medical student).

The statement above was made by a second year medical student in a "time-out" pause during a tutoring session with a standardized patient. The student was in the early part of an encounter with an angry SP mother whose daughter she suspected had received birth control pills from this "doctor". Seconds before the "time-out", or pause in interaction, the student had responded in a defensive and indignant tone almost matching the mother's, regarding her ethic of patient confidentiality. She was red faced and at a loss for words. I was struck by the student's explanation for her experience of being emotionally overwhelmed.

I am facilitating this session and as an observer have been watching the student in her exchange with the SP become increasingly agitated over the course of the first few minutes of the encounter. During the pause, I listen to her talk about her struggles to remain organized, about what she thinks she missed (information) and what she would like to do next when she "goes back in". We talk about the mother's anger, and techniques the student might use to "de-escalate" the anger such as active listening techniques, - acknowledgement, open ended questions…, and this is when she apologizes for her amygdala. What makes this explanation possible?

I contend that this entire educational experience is made possible by discourses that define emotion as neuro-biologically rooted and which can only be mastered through skills of practiced behavioural control. The student, the standardized patient, and I as a non-clinician teacher, are each implicated in reproducing an understanding of emotion as a set of interpersonal techniques performed to manipulate affect for the purposes of achieving "appropriate" professional behaviour. The student identifies her amygdala - a physical structure inside her head - as accounting for her "out of control" behaviour excusing herself from responsibility for her behaviour on the grounds that as she says she "is just wired this way". Yet the context, (practice with a difficult SP) and her apology, suggests that she believes that she should be able to (and is learning how to) control her emotional response through practice.

There is an elision of emotion and corporeality within medical education as it relates to the body of "the" physician. Physicians' "professional" white coated and contained bodies act as signifiers of physiological stasis. – not to be affected by turmoil. Such a stance isolates physicians, seeing that denial (of emotion) is needed collectively in order to reproduce its absence. The student in my example talks about her experience objectively – "my amygdala is out of control" – as if appealing to laws of generalization and causality. The being of them (emotion and affect) and the understanding of them are "through co-modification, inextricably connected by fast drying (calcified) ideological cement" (Newman, 1997, p. 125-6). They are an object to be fixed upon. The student claims her emotionality as a characteristic of her body. As Ahmed points out,

> Such thinking about emotion "is bound up with the securing of social hierarchy: emotions become attributes of bodies as a way of transforming what is 'lower' or 'higher' into bodily traits. Being emotional comes to be seen as universal and distinct from both personal and social contexts while at the same time, as a characteristic of some bodies and not others (Ahmed, 2004, p.4).

Thinking about emotion as physiological, psychological and inside us seems to foster multiple paradoxical readings. It is both universal – rooted in the universal 'body'– and distinctly personal. However, although universal, emotion discourses are also highly gendered with women being interpreted as the more emotional and less rational sex. As Lutz suggests, "It is opposed on the one hand, to the positively evaluated process of thought and, on the other hand, to a negatively evaluated estrangement from the world. To say that someone is 'unemotional' is either to claim that the person is calm, rational and deliberate or that he or she is withdrawn or uninvolved, alienated or even catatonic" (Lutz, 2007, p. 21). This tension shows up in such ideas as "detached concern" as a desired state for physicians perpetuated in exchanges and feedback practices with SPs, while diagnosable as depression or a psychiatric symptom in a patient. Alternative readings of emotion by (Ahmed, 2004; Boler, 1999; Hochschild, 2003; Lutz & Abu-Lughod, 1990; Kemper, 1993; Williams. 2001) regard emotions as social and cultural practices that do not belong inside bodies only but "form a social presence" (Ahmed, 2004, p.10), that circulates between bodies shaping them as effects of its circulation. Ahmed writes about the political and cultural work emotions do in shaping ideas and enactments which get projected onto bodies – "some bodies but not others" (Ahmed, 2004, p. 170). This work of projecting emotion "onto bodies of others not only works to exclude others from the realms of thought and rationality but, but also works to conceal the emotional aspects of thought and reason" (2004, p. 170). Such a reading of emotion and affect provides a helpful lens through which to examine the material implications different ideas about emotion have for patient care, medical student training and practicing medical professionals.

The student in my story was self-diagnosing not self-reflecting. She was locating her trouble with the SP inside herself as a physiological response that she seemed to suggest needed fixing (with medication or therapy?), not as something that occurred between their bodies and connected to a larger question of professionalism and an ethics of confidentiality. Her response was in effect telling me that she needed help for her amygdala, not that she didn't understand what was happening in this situation. The first view I contend shuts down educational possibilities while the second view opens them up. As a teacher in this setting her explanation diverted my attention from the fact that her anger arose as a result of a social interaction and appropriately as a response to her budding ethical awareness as a clinician. Her response did not need to be fixed or explained away. As well, her anger did not just happen to her, but between us all offering us an opportunity to learn through a particular instance about the crucial place of emotion in clinical thinking and interaction. Affect is integral to this conversation as it is also circulating as a force between bodies creating particular effects in their movement. Despite differences between them, emotion, body, mind and affect correspond in crucial ways in educational settings.

3.2.2 Gender/ Bodies/Emotion and Medical Professionalism

There is a well established feminist interrogation of the relationship between reason and emotion and its gendered political consequences (Boler 1999; Jaggar,1989; Spelman, 1982; Campbell, 1994; Lloyd, 1989; Bartky, 1998). In *Privilege in the Medical Academy* (1997), Delese Wear asks whether despite increased numbers of women in the academy "socialization processes are so powerful and profound that even now, critically massed women in medicine assume a colonizing role themselves, participate in the surveillance and quality control of novices into the profession and see that medicine makes a man out of every aspiring doctor? (1997, p. 105). The message is that emotions are not appropriate epistemic sources in medicine and in fact are "improper and disruptive responses in medical settings" (1997, p.107). Wear continues,

> By moulding the emotional character of young physicians-in-training in particular ways, medicine helps to guarantee its own reproduction, its own scripts and its own masks. It does so not by coercive force; rather 'it surveys, supervises, observes, measures the body's behavior and interactions with others...punish[ing] this resistant to its rule and forms (1997, p. 107).

Wear is describing a hegemonic power relation between professionalism and emotion which a view of competence as a form of knowledge maintains. Hegemony as a practice of power works largely though ideas as a way of representing the order of things to appear universal, natural, and synonymous with reality itself.

As described by Alison Jaggar; "Western epistemology has tended to view emotion with suspicion and even hostility" (Jaggar, 1989, p. 161). She continues,

> Reason has been associated with members of dominant political, social and cultural groups and emotion with members of subordinate groups. Prominent among those subordinate groups in society are people of colour, except for supposedly 'inscrutable oriental's and women (Jaggar, 1989, p.163-64).

To become a doctor is to become a detached, reasoned scientist and male. A view of the more pervasive exclusions made possible by rationalist epistemology is expressed by Anna Yeatman. (1994)

> Individuals who belong to groups which are consistently objectified by modern science – women, blacks, colonials, peasants and other groups…are admitted to the club only as exceptions to the norm for their group…They are admitted to the scientific club only if they combine an appropriate training in the procedures of foundationalist science with the adoption of the persona of the rationalist sovereign subject. However if on occasion they should contravene the scientific norms of disembodied, detached proceduralism and commit an emotional excess of some kind, this will be forgiven as an inevitable flaw which confirms their status as somewhat less than real scientists – subaltern scientists. The flaw is even required. (Yeatman 1994 p. 189-90 cited in Wear, 1997, p. 5).

This applies for women in varying roles in medicine: those who are teachers and deemed carriers of emotion and affect as knowledge to medical students, as well as to female medical students themselves who struggle with maintaining a body in control, already inscribed as the "wrong" body" (Wear, 1997). In my exchange with the female medical student her struggle to "get a grip" on her anger as part of her professional performance reproduces dominant values that reinforce basic social divisions based on gendered notions of professionalism. The fact that the student's emotion was anger is at least more acceptable than that of sadness or more explicitly anything that might make a professional cry. Cited as an "outlaw emotion" by Alison Jaggar (1989) crying in instances that are "conventionally inexplicable" is at the very least a sign that something is wrong and a strong indication of a power relation in which subordinated individuals are paying a disproportionately high price for maintaining the *status quo* (p. 166). "Crying is raw emotion, a body unable to control itself, internally externalized" (Cassells, 1996, p. 43).

With respect to bodies, as bell hooks argues, "Only the person who is most powerful has the privilege of denying their body" (hooks, 1994, p. 137). "The erasure of the body encourages us to think that we are listening to neutral, objective facts, facts that are not particular to who is sharing the information" (1994, p. 139). Pointing up power relations at the centre of medical professionalism, hooks' brings our attention to the imbalance between the body of the doctor which is pure (white coat) and at best invisible and the patient's which is the product of the medical gaze. While the physician's body is assumed to be healthy, (at least germ free) and in control of itself both physically and emotionally, the patient's body, is assumed to be "unwell" or "fragile" and out of control. The fragility is sexualized as it is women who are historically identified as having weaker physical and moral constitutions[1] in need of disciplinary medicinal support. Further differences between the bodies of professionals and their patients or trainees for that matter are class inflected with respect to bodily movement. Not only does this refer to patients' possible physical pain and symptomotology, but also to the idea that persons in the master professions (medicine, law) move less as they rely on "mind " and rationality while the majority of those for whom they tend may do physical work, labour or serve with their bodies.

"The standardizing impulses of modernity and the positivism of science" (Shildrick, 2002, p. 23) are still at work within medicine, with emotion dichotomously constructed as an object of empirical and evidence based on natural order and scientific scrutiny (neuroscience) as well as a Christian ethics and morality. A Western trained medical trainee is subject to individualizing discourses that recognize emotional alignment within moral, Christian parameters. At the same time the professionalizing project requires the erasure of emotion in order to ensure that objectivity and rationality prevail. The following section outlines an emotional intelligence framework which has become a technology though which strategies that perpetuate isolation, burn out, "disruptive" behaviour, and increased incidence of mental health addiction problems intersect with educational mandates.

3.3   Emotional Intelligence and Medical Education

The following section examines Emotional Intelligence (E.I.) as the dominant, contemporary assemblage through which emotion is understood and addressed in Western medical training popularized in the mid-nineties through the work of Daniel Goleman (1995). It is the most hegemonic framework supporting emotion as a skill to which we are all exposed both personally and professionally on a day-to-day basis. Teasing apart the ways in which an "emotion-as-skills" approach produces and reproduces what Deleuze and Guattari refer to as a "royal science apparatus", allows me to make visible how this mode of knowledge production constitutes relations and their material effects. Emotion is constructed as a "problem to be fixed", with empathy conceived of as both, ability and internal trait. "How do we stop the rot?" (Spencer, 2004, p. 916) was how one medical educator framed the problem, suggesting that there is a moral failure in medical trainees which can be addressed through professional training. The answer E.I. models suggest is to improve communication skills through practice and demonstration and to proliferate practices that produce what Deleuze and Guattari identify as an arborescent model of thought which they describe as a "tree logic" of reproduction.

"Arborescent systems are hierarchical systems with centres of signification and subjectification, central automata like organized memories (Deleuze & Guattari, 1987, p.16).

> Its goal is to describe a de facto state, to maintain balance in intersubjective relations, or to explore an unconscious that is already there from the start, lurking in the deep recesses of memory and language (1987, p.12).

This returns me to the idea of emotion constructed as a universal system of largely unconscious forces that act as internal signals. Within medicine this model of thought has political and material effects, for example with respect to ideas about standards of practice and emotional competency as a skill. It also has implications for those practicing medicine, their patients and the shape of profession as a whole.

3.3.1 Models of Emotional intelligence

The concept Emotional Intelligence was popularized by Daniel Goleman in his 1995 best seller *Emotional intelligence: Why it can matter more than IQ,* however, the term was first published by Peter Salovey and John Mayer in a journal entitled *Imagination, Cognition and Personality* in 1990. Previous to Salovey and Mayer the term "emotional intelligence" is traceable to a doctoral dissertation by Wayne Payne in 1986 which was never published (Payne, 1986).

Salovey and Mayer's version of emotional intelligence is based on a four branch model: 1) perception of emotion (in self and others); 2) assimilation of emotion to facilitate thought; 3) understanding emotion; and 4) managing and regulation of emotion in self and others, operationalizing the model as an 'abilities measure" (Ashkanazy&Daus, 2005, p.442). It is an arborescent cognitive-behavioural model that views "emotion perception" at the most rudimentary skill level while "emotion management" as the most complex. It is meant to differentiate between individuals in their emotion skills and abilities. The authors do not contend, like their predecessors, that beyond possible personality styles there is any physiological or specific neurological component involved in emotional intelligence.

Daniel Goleman has built a corporate empire out of emotional intelligence, expanding it into a comprehensive machine for organizational management and business leadership including motivational seminars on "Primal Leadership". "Emotional Intelligence" is a product line sold world wide in the form of measurement guides, self help books, online tools and which now includes a similar line of services and products for individuals interested in developing "social intelligence". His model combines skills, abilities, personality traits, and uniquely, rationalizes different emotional competencies such as emotional management along physiological lines. Emotional management for instance involves the amygdale or other "emotion centres" (Goleman, 1995, p. 19). He bases his claims on the neuro-scientific discoveries of Joseph Ledoux (1996) and Antonio Damasio (1994). Goleman clusters competencies related to emotional intelligence under four domains: self-awareness, self-management, social awareness, and relationship management. Each domain is described with accompanying abilities. For example, the self-management domain includes the competency of trust worthiness, and individuals who demonstrate this competency are authentic and reliable. There is a strong critical reaction to Goleman's capitalist enterprise from within academia. However it does not seem to have reduced the popularity of E.I. for possible use in everything from medical school admissions processes (Carrothers, 2000), to studies looking at the possible relationship between E.I. attributes and student's clinical skills as assessed by standardized patients (Elam, Stratton, et al, 2001).

Following Goleman a doctoral student, Reuven Bar-On, (1997) adapted measures he created for his dissertation on psychological well being according to Goleman's work. He includes positive qualities and conceptually slippery outcomes such as 'happiness' and 'self actualization' in his model. Bar-On's scales are branded EQ-I, "a multidimensional questionnaire measure of emotional intelligence now marketed and distributed by Multi-Health Systems" (Bar-On, 1997). His model consists of five broad domains and associated skills and like Goleman includes personality traits. Skills such as the ability to: assert one self, be empathic, control impulses and problem solve are divided into the four separate domains suggesting a refined system of differentiation. The final domain, general mood, is described by Bar-On as a facilitator of emotional intelligence and includes optimism and happiness.
(http://www.eiconsortium.org/measures/eqi.html)

In summary, these E.I. models suggests that it is possible to objectively determine correct responses on a scale, which assumes that there is a correct answer to be had. All three models assume that emotional intelligence is a unique entity that does not overlap with other constructs such as mental ability or personality. Most interesting is the presumption that something called emotional intelligence actually exists and is not simply a fabricated construct serving administrative rather than educational or therapeutic ends.

3.3.2 Emotional Intelligence: Main Ideas

The main ideas produced within an Emotional Intelligence (E.I.) framework in medical education are: Emotion is inside the individual's brain and needs to be made visible in order to be known; emotion is the individual's professional responsibility; emotions are self directed and other directed skills to be learned through practice. In medical education it is possible to assess emotion as a skill or attribute through observation. Finally, emotions are unpredictable and need to be fixed, managed or regulated. These ideas are contingent on each other. Invisible professional attributes such as empathy, need to be transformed into visible entities in order to be observed. Such concepts as "detached concern" get taken up along with empathy as an arbiter of emotional engagement and rational distance. Both empathy and detached concern will be discussed in more detail in a later section.

Emotion as a skill and ability belonging to an individual requires it be performed – a specific kind of performance which is instrumental and meant to demonstrate rather than evoke as in other kinds of performance. Assessment of individual performances of emotion may occur in standardized settings and employ psychometric calculations to determine an individual's placement within a normative range. Particular and peculiar observer and performer subject positions and technologies are produced through this activity. The rationale is that emotion and affect get in the way of clear thinking and objective decision making, producing effects that are unpredictable, beyond our control and which need to be managed.

Within this psychological construction concepts of "intelligence" and "emotions" converge along a trajectory related to ideas about ability, skills acquisition and performance. Standardized patients become visible as a technology for teaching and assessing "communications skills", "empathy", "compassion", and "professional attitudes". Such notions as "patient centred" and more recently "relationship centred" clinical method, rapport, empathy, verbal and non verbal behaviour, and self reflection, all observable and measurable psychometrically, are produced, creating both resistances and positivities. Desire, as a productive force in the creation of new knowledges, becomes tethered to observable relational matrices; what Deleuze and Guattari identify as molar segmentarities. Molar segmentarities describe a system that is rigid proscribed and brittle with a tendency to break. Ideas about the interiority and uniqueness of an individual's emotion and thoughts produces subject positions, for example, the authorized interpreter (in this case teacher) of the interior other and the subject who authorizes such knowing and interpretation (student, patient). Implied is a direct causal relationship between emotion and affect – "My anger makes me behave in a particular way" – that is then remediable. Boundary tensions are put into play related to vying professionalization projects related to standardized patients as: scholars, non clinical teachers, simulation coaches, communication specialists, and facilitators. Questions about definitions of performance/simulation and the place of related pedagogies for educational purposes are made possible.

3.3.4 Achieving Emotional Competency

According to Goleman's E.I. model we can interpret the medical student's comment about her amygdala as reflecting a personal physiological weakness that she needs to correct through psychological means in order to achieve empathic competency. "Competency" is of central importance to medical professionalism. As a construct it is tied to Deleuze and Guattari's idea of "tracing" which as an activity is reproductive, redundant and closed. "The map has to do with performance whereas the tracing always involves alleged "competence" (Deleuze & Guattari, 1987, p.12-13). Competence they suggest "...confines every desire and statement to a genetic axis or overcoding structure, and makes infinite, monotonous tracings of the stages on that axis or the constituents of that structure" (Deleuze & Guattari, 1987, p.13). Tracing is a product of arborescent or tree logic, more interested in the points of arrival or outcome than in the line between them. SPs function as what Deleuze and Guattari call a war machine[3] when they are coded as tools for the purposes of developing practitioner competence as a point in fact and not along a line of connection.

My configuration of student, SP, teacher in the story at the beginning of the chapter is an arborescent model that traces a capitalist neo-liberal machine, producing needs, while co-modifying internal attributes in order to generate capital in the form of self-help training and E.I. type improvement modules. The unit of analysis is the individual and their internal workings, not the multiplicity of becomings in the room. Emotion becomes a discreet entity essentially attached to, but less than, rationality. This separation works to reify dichotomies of gender, race, culture that are assumed to be true and real. In other words there is one right way to be emotional or at least a right range of emotion for professional purposes. These get reified in both visible and invisible daily practices, for example, the College of Physicians and Surgeons of Ontario regulatory designation of "disruptive doctor" (Policy Statement #4-07 College of Physicians and Surgeons of Ontario).

Deleuze and Guattari distinguish between "desiring productions" as those assemblages that create becomings and multiplicities and "social productions" as those forces that can only trace or what is already established or known (Deidrich, 2007, p. 191). E.I. represents a "social production" which can only trace or reproduce what is already established with regards to medicine's hegemonic binary logic.

3.3.5 E.I. Models and Measurement

These authors have developed and marketed the measurement aspects of their work within the academic community as well as to business and popular audiences. The U.S. military now offer EI programs to build "resilience" in soldiers in order to help them prepare for and pre-empt the trauma of battle! Salovey and Mayer have a one hundred and forty-one item *Mayer-Salovey Carruso Emotional Intelligence Test (MSCEIT)*. Goleman's scale the *Emotional Competency Inventory (ECI)* is a self report and 360 degree assessment although there are different versions of it with varying numbers of competencies arrayed in different clusters of skills – "one with twenty-five competencies arrayed in five clusters, another with twenty-one competencies in four clusters" (Boyatzis, 2000 cited in Lewis, 2005, p. 346). Bar-On's measurement tool is a self report one hundred and thirty-three item scale.

Even within an arborescent model of thought there are conceptual problems with the construction of emotion as a stable measureable object.

Psychometrically, the scales requiring self report responses assume that: 1.) Emotion is a stable and unchanging object to be measured, 2.) An individual has insight into what this might look or feel like. 3.) It is possible to accurately assess one's own performance based on unique knowledge of one's emotional workings, and, 4.) The scales are designed to assess an individual's perceived rather than "real" emotional intelligence. Tests that are not self report, like Salovey and Mayer's MSCEIT (1990) suffer from assumptions about the objective simplicity and normativity of the construct being measured. A person is asked to respond to different images or statements on a five point Likert scale. The scoring is based on how most people would answer, as if the responses are generalizeable, making it "objectively" possible to determine correct responses based on a standard mean.

3.3.6 Emotional Intelligence: Products and Practices in Medical Education

The co-modification of emotion is one of the most productive effects of an E.I. discourse within medical education. Emotion constructed as skills and abilities fits into medicine's culture of accountability in which individual performances are amenable to educative processes and professional regulation. The focus is on outcomes and emerging professionals as reliable products. It is once again a neoliberal discourse which places the onus for achievement of emotional "competence" on the individual, eliding power relations embedded in educational and regulatory mandates as well as investment by the State[4] in a manageable populace. In this assemblage emotions are cognitive processes while behaviours are evidence of an internal response to social and environmental factors. A medical student's empathy or altruistic sensibility can be right or wrong as measured on a multiple choice questionnaire or plotted onto a checklist during an observed performance with an SP, as if an individual's "values, attitudes and behaviours" represent a single, de-contextualized, observable assemblage.

As such E.I is what Deleuze and Guattari refer to as a State apparatus. As Deleuze and Guattari's theory of the State suggests, E.I. works in the interest of the State.

> Theirs is the discourse of sovereign judgment, of stable subjectivity, legislated by "good" sense, of rock like identity, "universal" truth, and (white male justice." "Thus the exercise of their thought is in conformity with the aims of the real State, with the dominant significations and with the requirements of the established order" (Deleuze, 1977, p. 20 cited by Massumi, in Deleuze & Guattari, 1987, p.ix).

Taken up until recently largely within in the business profession by corporate management, leadership and organizational behaviour groups as a methodology for achieving success in personal and professional endeavours, medical education since the 1980's has grown increasingly interested in adopting its methods. As a set of psychologically derived ideas E.I. meets medicine's humanistic goals of developing caring professionals while providing a dependable method for measuring and judging capacities seen as not amenable to reliable capture. Capture of emotion in this kind of a system calls for a specific unidirectional and grid like movement. Medical trainees can be directed into specific performances (OSCEs) that in focusing on outcomes exclude creative processes, widened webs of relationships, and ways of thinking and adapting. Learning is a rhizomatic activity following non linear movement that begins in the middle and operates in qualitatively unique space in which there are changes in direction, intensities and speeds in response to desire as a force. An E.I. model of learning can not recognize such ambiguity and uncertainty of outcome.

A shift that took place in capitalist societies of the late twentieth century has moved us from mechanisms of discipline to ones of control. This movement, identified by Deleuze and others, has extended from bio-politics: Foucault's disciplinary production of subjects whose behaviours express internalized social norms and are focused at the level of the population, in order to control societies "aimed at a never ending modulation of moods, capacities, affects, potentialities..." (Clough, 2007, p. 17). Within an E.I. rationale we can see how "pre-individual bodily capacities are made the site of capital investment for the realization of profit – not only in terms of bio-technology, bio-medicalization, and genetics but also in terms of a technologically dispersed education/training in self-actualization and self control at the pre-individual, communal, national, and trans national levels" (Clough, 2007, p. 21).

3.4 Emotion: a problem to be fixed

> Those feelings just get in the way. They don't fit, and I'm going to learn to get rid of them. Don't know how yet and some of the possibilities are scary (Second Year female).

This quote is from a study conducted by Allen Smith and Sherry Kleinman (1989, p. 68) which explored medical student strategies for managing their emotions during early training experiences with the human body–living and dead. The authors found through two years of participant observation that a hidden curriculum of unspoken rules and resources for dealing with unwanted emotions encouraged students to develop distancing and rationalizing strategies that reproduced "the perspective of modern Western medicine and the kind of doctor-patient relationship it implies." (Smith &Kleinman, 1989, p. 56).

Dominant models for understanding emotion within clinical medicine suggest that both the experience and expression of emotion are problematic in practice. Framed as dangerous, unpredictable, beyond one's control, and something that needs to be trained, it is separated from rationality – on the other side of the Cartesian divide. Emotion gets in the way, overwhelming reason and possibly leading to dangerous decisions and actions and needs to be evacuated from the rational in order for clinicians to function successfully as professionals. Discourses of emotion which see it as a form of intelligence or set of physiological traits are supported by medicine's rational, scientific, objective, and empirical ontology. The word "emotion" does not appear in the many regulatory and accreditation documents (Association of American Medical Colleges, Accreditation Council for Medical Education, Can MEDS, Educating Future Physicians of Ontario, College of Family Physicians of Canada, College of Physicians and Surgeons of Ontario) despite its existence as a social force that needs to be controlled. Emotion in fact is replaced in professional documents by the term, "attitudes" which is more easily measureable. Boler suggests that "By the end of the second World War, the social sciences were increasingly focused on measurement and the study of attitudes which could be shaped through social control more easily than emotions. It is a rationalist version of behaviour modification and social control" (Boler, 1997, p. 213). The way in which emotion as an object of study is framed has potentially unintended effects such as painting them as a problem which needs to be fixed.

There is an exquisite relationship between ideas about rationality which reinforce professional authority, and the titration of amount and type of emotion permitted in the practice of medicine. As professionals "Doctors are supposed to treat all patients alike (that is well) regardless of personal attributes, and without emotions that might disrupt the clinical process or the doctor-patient relationship" (Smith and Kleinman, 1989, 56). Strategies to help students achieve appropriate professional ideals of "affective neutrality" (Parsons 1951) and "detached concern" (Lief and Fox, 1963) rest on particular gendered ideas about emotion and its relationship to rationality, cognition and behaviour.

3.4.1 Emotion as Demonstration of Skill

Within medical education currently and heath professional education more broadly, emotion is being incorporated into research along a number of paths. For example, cognitive neuroscientists are exploring the effect of the release of different neuro- chemicals such as cortisol in stressful situations and its effect on practitioner behaviour (Leblanc, 2010). Research is being carried out on the effect of emotion on learning and retention of information as well as on practitioner situational awareness. As mentioned at the beginning of the chapter with respect to clinical training, one set of research focuses on emotion as a kind of performance and explores ways to improve emotional competence through practical applications of communication skills. Another approach sees emotion as a quasi-cognitive tool and pays attention to increasing trainees' abilities to recognize emotion in self and others, over the practical aspects of how to communicate it. The various assemblages created in these different approaches focus on performances or demonstrations of emotion that surface individual interior traits or behaviours. I suggest that this is a slight of hand that appropriates performance as a form of demonstration or outcome in order to reiterate and reproduce rational order.

A "demonstration" is a particular kind of performance which is instrumental not evocative as other kinds of performance may be. For example, medical trainees are observed in acts of demonstrating competency in the skill of suturing (the example provided in the guide). It can be assessed for both the performance of technique and success of outcome. The same rationale exists for demonstrating emotion as a skill. For example, empathy or compassion as a demonstration is reduced in complexity to a uni-directional movement. To demonstrate is to focus on the activity of "doing to" an "other" and valuing what is observable as an outcome – the effect of the competency (calmer, more compliant patient, or colleague), while not acknowledging the contingent, messy and ambiguous affective dimensions of the undertaking. In this disconnected realm, empathy as a demonstration can easily be carried out as a manipulation and normalizing task.

Practicing empathy as a communication skill with standardized patients has this potential. Hanna and Fins (2006), writing about the effect of altered power relations in simulated patient teaching, suggest:

> A medical student may, through practice in simulation encounters, be able to master all the skills and tricks of surface communication and be able to use them very effectively in an OSCE and in later practice effectively. .[But] Does he or she ever learn to master the discursive

and ontological power that makes the physician-patient relationship an invigorated, productive lived reality rather than a set of acting techniques (p. 267).

An outcomes approach which suggests human connection can be learned and assessed as a demonstration of technique may be creating new realities where the performed comes to stand in for the "real" and define it in new ways. Such possibilities are supported by performance examinations like OSCEs in which the pressure to dissimulate or act that which is not present, as well as, to simulate, performing "as if" one cared, according to standardized checklists, results in pretend empathy, demonstrations of diagnostic thinking and management. As Hodges (2009) reported, one student told him that "the only time that I feel like [I am] faking is when [I] try to be empathic. It is odd, I think, to express empathy to somebody when you know they don't really have the condition" (p. 127). I think this speaks beautifully to the confusion about the "doing: that medical students are expected to demonstrate. It is a narcissistic closed loop that involves the "other" only instrumentally, in the achievement of the goal of demonstrating ones competence. I am not suggesting that this student needs to "feel" for someone who is not really ill. But I think what is odd is that the possibility of feeling is linked to an idea about what is real about what he is doing, and not to the exchange itself. Why did the student have to act as if he cared? Whose expectation was he pretending to meet and for what purpose?

The role of standardized patients as a tool in this discussion intersects with ideas of reality, performance, and possibilities that emerge from their unique location within circumstances in which emotion as a skill is being taught and assessed. They are caught in the same web as the students, enacting "appropriate" intensities and types of responses according to expectations about student needs, and the medical profession's ideas about patients.

3.4.2 Implications of an E.I. Assemblage in Medical Education Training

An emotional intelligence assemblage within medical education has implications for the profession, the health professional and the medical trainee not to mention the patient. Emotion defined as individualized and private leads to increased student and practitioner isolation and burn out. Universalizing emotion as a physiological phenomenon erases the socio cultural impact of different ideas of emotion from the educational landscape. Emotions identified as outside the norm of acceptable remain hidden to be handled individually by "getting control of oneself," or "putting feelings aside". Such thinking embedded in curricula and regulatory documents maintains a conception of the individualistic learning models. Accountability strategies that centre on the emotion skills and abilities of the individual make invisible the situated inequities and material pressures which shape a work place. Emotion seen as static and tied to internal physiology, rather than complex and part of a dynamic cultural process constrains possibilities for addressing the very problems such an approach produces.

It seems that there is a right and wrong way to experience and demonstrate emotion as a medical professional. Judgments are made possible by technologies that support systems of observation and surveillance. Psychometrics, highly formalized performance / demonstration protocols, observation guides and performance checklists, assessment and feedback, video and digital technology and standardized patients are provided with authority. The ways in which one participates in this assemblage includes SPs as teachers, acting coaches, and in some cases assessors, students as performers, and clinicians as expert observers, all legitimized and granted authority by constructing the invisible as something that needs to be regulated and managed. Such assemblages are not only subject to power relations but are also shaped by desire.

Assemblages of desire are another way of looking at emotional engagement that moves us beyond the ideas that isolate emotion as internal and instrumental. As compositions that are essentially passional, assemblages connect us to each other through relationships that create new rationalities or ways of looking at and producing things. Such an analysis suggests emotion is affective, and, increased receptivity and capacity for action are possible through qualitative shifts. In such a view desire is a productive force of becomings that are immanent in all relations.

In the following section I examine empathy as the most esteemed of emotions in medical training and practice and the ideas that inform it. Affect in this writing is understood as emotional expression and not in its more elaborated ontological form which will be described further in the section following. It is no surprise that emotional intelligence ideas in the form of cognitive behavioural influences are visible in education related to empathy. As an object of focus within medical training, empathy sits at an intersection of morality, ethics and professionalism and is attached to ideas of competency all of which need to be made observable and measureable.

3.5   Empathy

Empathy can be seen as the privileged and most visible site of medicine's concern regarding the status of emotion in the profession and its moral failure to produce "good" humanistic doctors. As I have described, the literature on empathy includes foundational articles on "detached concern", studies of cognitive abilities and traits related to "awareness and understanding emotion in self and other" as well as the demonstration of empathy as a skill.

3.5.1 Empathy as Detached Concern

> As imperturbability is largely a bodily endowment, I regret to say that there are those amongst you, who, owing to congenital defects may never be able to acquire it. Education will however do much; and with practice and experience the majority of you may except to attain to a fair measure (Osler, 1904, p.4).

In William Osler's (1849-1914) famous valedictorian address to the graduating class of the University of Pennsylvania school of Medicine in 1889 the idea of "aequanimitas", or equanimity was put forth as a professional necessity. "Imperturbability" stood for the bodily virtue of calmness or "a judicious measure of obtuseness" (1889, p. 4), while "Aequanimitas" stood for the complimentary mental virtue of composure and acceptance with respect to the hardships that come with life and the practice of medicine" (1889, p. 5). However he advises, "This should not lead to hardness in dealing with patients" (1889, p. 6). Osler encouraged the medical graduates to develop the other gentlemanly virtues of courage, patience and honour. The idea was that detachment and calm are empathic and necessary for a full and accurate understanding of a patient's problem. The tension between emotional engagement and rational detachment describes medicine's definition of empathy as "detached concern". Integral to a code of professionalism as ethical and moral undertaking, the issue of how much emotion is too much and how it should best be performed professionally is couched in cognitive behavioural terms with effects on patients, health professionals, the profession, and ultimately medical trainees.

3.5.2 Effect on Medical Trainees

> The empathic physician is sufficiently detached or objective in his attitude toward the patient to exercise sound medical judgment and keep his equanimity, yet he also has enough concern for the patient to give him sensitive, understanding care. This set of attitudes has been termed by one of us (R.C.F.) detached concern (Lieff & Fox, 1963, 12).

The rationale echoes Osler's description of "aequanimitas" and suggests emotion gets in the way of sound medical judgment needing to be proscribed for the safety and benefit of the patient. In a study entitled *Affect and Its Control in the Medical Intern* (Daniels 1960), the author studied different "modes" of affective involvement and mechanisms of its control between interns and patients. The affective involvement was graded in intensity from "(1) an almost compete lack of any affective involvement; (2) somewhat intellectualized understanding of the problem of his patient, an appreciation of his intrinsic value and the personal implications of his illness and suffering, together with a disinterested service on behalf of all whose illness leads them to help; to (3) a complete emotional identification in which the intern empathically suffers a great deal" (p. 259). "It is the definition in category two that is explicitly prescribed by the medical system" (p. 260). Affective deviation in either direction – either toward indifference to the patient as a person or over involvement emotionally with patient or family - are discouraged within system for the sake of the patient. The author observes that inclination toward less affective involvement is sanctioned however as it is supported by the demands of a more specialized disciplinary knowledge and skill base i.e. surgery, which in the end will benefit the patient. The interns in the study internalized the ethos of "detached concern as a necessity realizing "the deleterious effect of profuse sympathy upon the patient's welfare" (Daniels, 1960, p. 263). As one intern noted, "When sympathy is too profuse, the patient becomes suspicious that that is all you have to offer" (p.263). It seems that caring too much for patients' limits professional authority and can interfere with patient care. The norms related to affective neutrality are strong in medicine with evacuation of emotion from reason considered a professional necessity. The study reifies the idea of detached concern as a normalizing technology through its classificatory approach effectively reproducing a dichotomy which as described earlier devalue emotion and affect.

Writing on the problem of empathy and its decline in medical students takes many forms. The E. I. literature directs our attention to statistical studies locating the problem inside the individual student as a product of the medical school curriculum (Satterfield & Hughes, 2007). Empathy scales are put to work measuring longitudinally the changes in individuals' feelings and behaviours. These measurements suffer the conceptual and practical problems identified earlier however there is large scale uptake of a cognitive and behavioural approach to emotion within medical education proliferating studies across the breadth of medical school. It is an accepted truth that medical trainees lose idealism and become cynical over the course of their training and many fault the lack of healthy role modeling and the informal experiences or "hidden curriculum" in this regard (Rabow, 2010; Hafferty. 2000). Under great pressure to prove themselves worthy of entering the profession, students are afraid to admit that they have uncomfortable feelings about patients or procedures and hide these feelings behind a cloak of competence (Smith &Kleinman, 1989, p. 57). Moving beyond an instrumental approach to empathy means that we engage it as a capacity that is as much about imagination as it is about skill or abilities. This allows opportunities for different kinds of inquiry, collective sharing and collaborative understanding.

3.5.3 Effect on the Medical Professional

> There is muted crying in bathrooms and stairwells all over the hospitals. The perception is that colleagues, patients and even friends see any breakdown as an indicator of not being a good doctor (Dr. Joy Albuquerque, Associate Medical Director of the physician health program, Ontario Medical Association, cited in Globe and Mail, June 26, 2007, L5).

The rationale suggests that "detached concern" needs to be in place in order to avoid physician burnout related to the day to day work of caring for patients. "Isolation, sadness at prolonged human tragedies, long hours of service, chronic lack of sleep, and depression at futile and often incomprehensible therapeutic manoeuvres turn even the most empathic of our children from caring physicians into tired terminators" (Spiro, 1993, cited in Spencer, 2004 p. 916-17). The statement reflects the onus placed on individual practitioners to cope by themselves with the emotional consequences of their work and the role of the profession as paternalistic guardians. Emotional work is a balancing act. Michael Evans (2007) writes "Doctors privately point out that the public is always calling for them to be more emotionally involved – yet only to a point. That there is a tipping point between the usual emotional give and take of friendship and the 'neutral scholar' that good doctors seem to balance" (Globe and Mail, L5).

Medical professionalism is a gendered discourse. Prevailing and deeply entrenched views of emotion as equated with the feminine weakness, and inconstancy, as opposed to strength, suggests to me as a reader that the person in the quote at the top of the section is a woman hiding in a stairwell struggling to cope. The idealizing definitions of empathy from Osler through to the present day are "heroic". They paint the image of a doctor as a man, an individual and sole upholder of standards struggling against all odds to maintain control of "himself" in order to serve mankind. The professional call for altruism masks a narcissism that isolates and glorifies the private suffering and sacrifice of the physician as individual and saviour. The ideas related to professional definitions of empathy have material implications for training and practice. Supported by an emotional intelligence discourse, accreditation, licensing and regulatory documents institutionalize and maintain this individualized and pseudo heroic version of professional agency as central to the practice of medicine.

3.5.4 Effect on the Patient

He lies on the couch unable to move, in pain, legs and scrotum swollen. Robert Skinner is in the end stages of bladder cancer and has agreed to see a visiting family doctor today at the request of his home care nurse who is very worried about him. She saw the book *The Final Exit*[5] on his coffee table the other day and is afraid that he is contemplating suicide. The family doctor who volunteers to visit with this patient is participating in a Saturday palliative care workshop. He is one of a group of practicing physicians from a range of disciplines who have identified end of life care as an area of interest and challenge. The patient is a standardized patient who like the man he is portraying is 75 years old.

Mr. Skinner is angry and sick of living in pain. He has decided that there is nothing more the doctors can do for him and he is ready to go. He doesn't want to see anyone – not his sister who lives in an assisted living apartment upstairs and is also very ill and can't move. He tells the doctor he has said goodbye to her and to everyone else who matters to him. The reason for the visit from the doctor's perspective is to see how Mr. Skinner is doing and to help with pain meds or in any other way that he can. Mr. Skinner's agenda is to ask if the doctor will assist him in killing himself. This is a real case and the request is something that the palliative care physicians tell us they deal with more than one would think.

The session is set up as a facilitated conversation so that the physician in the "hot seat" talking with Mr. Skinner is able to pause or "time-out" at any point and ask for help from his colleagues or those of us facilitating – myself and a palliative care physician.

This is an especially difficult situation for the interviewer because he is in front of his peers and because there are no right answers here. His approach, the decisions he makes and the words that he uses are not generalizable. And so he begins:

Doctor: Mr. Skinner, I am Dr Smith. I am replacing your doctor who is away right now. How are you doing today?

Mr. Skinner: What does it look like?

Doctor: Are you in pain? Your nurse tells me that she is worried about you?

Mr. Skinner: I'm in pain and I am sick of being here.

Doctor: What do you mean sick of being here?

Mr. Skinner: (angry) I am in pain, I can't move and I don't want to be living like this anymore.

Doctor: How has your mood been Mr. Skinner? Have you been depressed?

Mr. Skinner: No.

Doctor: How is your appetite? How are you sleeping? Is there anyone you like to visit with?

Mr. Skinner: No.

Doctor: What pain medications are you on?

Mr. Skinner: I don't know I just take the pills she gives me.

Doctor: Do you want to come into hospital? We can,,,

Mr. Skinner: No.

At this point the doctor pauses. He is aware that he is "missing something" but he can't figure out what it is or how to flush "it" out so that he can "deal with it". One of his colleagues suggests that he try to find out more about Mr. Skinner – What did he like to do when he was able to move around? Who was in his life that he might like to see at this point? Is there anything that he looks forward to? Doctor Smith goes back into the interview:

Doctor: What did you do for work Mr. Skinner?

Mr. Skinner: Regional manager of Loblaws. Damn good one.

Doctor: Is there anything that you look forward to over the course of a day?

Mr. Skinner: I look forward to not having to live like this.

Doctor: We can take care of your pain and make you more comfortable.

Mr. Skinner: I do not want to be more comfortable. I do not want your pity or your concern or more pain meds. You and the other doctors have done all that you can. You don't get it.

Doctor: We can arrange to have your sister come for a visit or have you go up and see her?

Mr. Skinner: I don't want anyone to see me like this, least of all my sister. She has enough troubles.

Doctor: I understand this is very difficult for you.

Mr. Skinner: (angry) Do you? Do you really understand what it is like to have someone wipe your bum, change your diapers? I am a grown man.

Doctor: Your life still has quality Mr. Skinner.

Mr. Skinner: You haven't heard a word I have said.

Doctor: Do you like hockey?

Mr. Skinner: Go away. Oh my God. Get out of here.

3.6. Witnessing: An alternative understanding

What is missing between them doesn't have to do with words spoken or not spoken. They are operating in different registers and have different agendas. The doctor wants to fix the unfixable and the patient wants to be heard – that his life is unlivable, and possibly to ask for help in ending his misery. There is no "fix" that anyone can provide. The doctor is saying many of the "right things" but he is still not able to "help" Mr. Skinner. How can this doctor sit with Mr. Skinner's suffering? Is it possible for him to engage this man from a place of not knowing, and practice a witnessing that acknowledges his pain without imposing his own solution on the "problem". What is passing between them is beyond words?

Lisa Diedrich calls this "practicing at a loss," "which would require that doctors give up the myth of control, acknowledge their failure to always have all the answers and to not turn away from suffering" (Diedrich, 2004, p. 157). Braidotti goes one step further suggesting the need for courage to sit on the edge of the abyss, look into it and let other forces come to the rescue" (Braidotti, 2006, p. 201). Such an undertaking however requires "compassion and fortitude to learn to see things differently, no matter how perilous the course for all involved" (Boler 1999, p. 176). At the core of such a critical approach is the task of questioning our own emotional investments as attachments to particular cultural and personal truths and to unsettle them. To see these as "inscribed habits of (in) attention" (Boler, 1999, p. 186), means to interrogate not only what one is assuming to be "truth" but to locate oneself historically and contingently as complicit in the very problems being addressed in the other's pain. "It is an invitation to move beyond self-reflection toward a collective witnessing that engages critically our role in the suffering that unfolds around us daily" (1999, p.

183). Central to this invitation to think and act differently is the idea of witnessing. Witnessing in contrast to spectating is a process in which "we do not have the luxury of seeing a static truth or fixed certainty. As a medium of perception, witnessing is a dynamic process and cannot capture meaning as a conclusion" (Felman, 1992, p. 5 cited in Boler 1999, 186).

The idea of witnessing resonates on a number of levels with my story of Mr. Skinner and the Doctor. It is important first of all for me as a facilitator in this situation to realize that we have all brought our histories and experiences into the room with us. To bring to the surface closely held and not always visible beliefs about what doctors are supposed to say and do, let alone feel, is risky territory. The doctor didn't say or do anything wrong. Why was the patient so angry? The doctor was perplexed that his words didn't work? There was something missing that the patient felt as dismissal. It happened in between the words, a failure to take seriously that which cannot be seen. The questions were rote – he wanted information and a solution and to be successful as the kind and wise physician. Unearthing this attachment to a narcissistic dream is not for me to push but possibly for us to arrive at together, maybe today, maybe not. As a non-clinician facilitator in this session recognizing that the most vulnerable person in the room is the doctor exploring new territory through an affective and emotional experience is important.

Deterritorializing and reterritorializing this exchange has nothing to do with the clinical realm of medications and hospitalizations, nor with communication skills. In fact it is a trap to frame this exchange in terms of the ethical question of assisted suicide – yes or no. This is an important aspect of the encounter with Mr. Skinner and pushes ethical, moral, emotional buttons, but in this conversation a hypothetical ethics stands in and gets employed to avoid practicing an ethics of engagement. We easily get stuck here as we shuffle from fact to opinion in order to avoid the more pressing conversation about suffering. What did the doctor and all of us together learn in the end? The patient experienced Doctor Smith's refusal to acknowledge his suffering as dismissal. There are no right words to say to make a situation like this better. Mr. Skinner is not going to feel better. There is a limit to what medical knowledge and this doctor can "solve". We are, in the end, left with a question and a problem, not an answer or solution. Deleuze suggests that we are in nomad territory. "The very notion of the 'problem' is related to the war machine" (Deleuze & Guattari 1987, p.365). "Whereas the theorem belongs to the rational order, the problem is affective and is inseparable from the metamorphosis, generations and creations within science itself" (Deleuze & Guattari 1987, p.362). What does it mean to acknowledge our powerlessness as human beings in the face of suffering? As a teacher for whom emotion and affect are the vehicle for learning, I question what knowledge is being constructed when such questions are left unexplored?

3.7   Affect

> Affects and emotions flow and crash upon meanings as rivers violently cross and carve the surfaces of the earth and rock (Boler, 1996, p.24).

There are many and varied contributions within the humanities, social sciences and the clinical and natural sciences to debates about what affect is, how it is related to emotion and ultimately what emotion and affect do politically and socially as forces that shape and are shaped by our day to day practices. "Affect functions differently to emotion; affect is inassimilable and hence exists outside the assemblage over-coded by rationality" (Boler, 1996, p. 11). There is often a conflation of affect with emotional expression, confounding understanding about their differences as well as their complex relationship to each other. "Affect constitutes a non-linear complexity out of which narration of conscious states such as emotion are subtracted but always with a never to be conscious autonomic remainder" (Clough, 2007, p. 2). From this perspective emotion is the capture of affective movement made conscious and named.

Within the medical sciences affect refers to expressions (gestures movements, dress and thought patterns) delineated as part of a pathological picture. In a medical education framework, emotion embodied by SPs is seen as a set of practices constructed and performed according to particular social and political arrangements. Affect in this context is seen as supplemental information focused on communication skills. It is extrinsic to clinical content and is seen as an additional element. Encounters have words and phrases that are more or less effective and helpful but which are separate from the movement of affect and thought that occurs wordlessly. Creating and enacting patient roles necessitates affective fluidity between bodies, and between worlds in the course of performing individual stories. It is in this space that witnessing others suffering and joy occurs. Affect is slippery because it is always in excess of that which can be captured and named. It is always between, and in that instant if only a flash, it produces its own irreducibility. (Deleuze & Guattari, 1987). Deleuze sees affects as an essential feature of the war machine – weapons: "That fill a smooth space in the manner of a vortex with the possibility of springing up at any point" (1987, p. 381).

From a post structuralist perspective, the affective work in which SP teachers engage is an open-ended and ongoing exchange rather than an instrumental and objectified approach to learning as "skills acquisition" or as communication skills teaching and practice. For example, there is no entity or content in affect as understood by Deleuze and Guattari. It is not in a dialectical relationship with content but is ontologically its own entity. Affectivity is the force that aims at fulfilling a subject's capacity for interaction and freedom. "It is Spinoza's *conatus,* or the notion of *potentia* as the affirmative aspect of power" (Braidotti, 2006, p. 148).

3.7.1 Affect/Expression

The world does not exist outside its expression (Deleuze, 1993, 132, in Massumi, 2002, p. xiii).

For Massumi, affect is tied up with surfaces of expression. Expression is always an event and the event is everything (2002, p. 14). With respect to affect a break occurs in the direct correspondence between the saying and the said, with forms of content and forms of expression having their own materiality. He states, "Mediation steals centre stage from conformity and correspondence" (2002, p. xvi), "between the form of content and the form of expression there is only the process of *their passing into each other*, in other words of their immanence, of their mutual deterritorialization" (2002, p. xviii). It is an emergent and singular process in which the unexpected and the atypical expression is formed at the hinge between non-verbal and verbal expression. For Ahmed, as for Massumi; "The movement between signs and objects converts into affect" (Ahmed, 2004, p. 45). Similar to Boler she suggests that emotions do not positively inhabit *anybody* or *anything* meaning that the subject is simply one nodal point in the economy, rather than its origin or destination.

For Massumi, following on the work of Spinoza, Deleuze and Guattari, affect is the virtual co-presence of potentials (Zournazi, 2002). His argument is intricate in that he argues for what Foucault called "incorporeal materialism" a virtual space of becoming which is embodied yet exists in potential only and includes within it a Deleuzian ontology of "becoming" (Massumi,2002, p. 5). For Massumi the conversion of the surface distance into intensity is also the conversion of the materiality of the body into an event" (Massumi, 2002, p. 14). It is the material manifested as movement between bodies. For me this akin to an in drawn breath before an action or spoken word – a space filled with infinite possibility.

In these descriptions the distinction between affect and emotion seems to be one of different qualities and directions of movements, with emotion acting as a "socio linguistic fixing" and affect as the "unassimilabile" the escape, or that which "leaks out." It contaminates empirical space as unknowable and therefore resistant to critique.

> Affect is co extensive with the war machine. They are in relation to each other as "speed, vertical or swirling movement…" (Deleuze & Guattari, 1987, p. 381).

Capture of emotions and affect within the molar segmentarity of medical education takes place on many fronts, for example through the scripting of SP roles, their standardized performances and the practice of feedback about what the experience was like for the "becoming patient' experience of the SP. "It is as if the 'savants' of nomad science were caught between a rock and a hard place between the war machine that nourishes and inspires them and the State that imposes upon them the order of reason" (Deleuze & Guattari, 1987, p.362). The practice of "feedback" itself consists of a taxonomy of techniques, styles and attitudes that gets used heuristically as a short cut - a straight line between two points - in order to address the student's observed behaviours. Movement outside of this template can lead to disciplinary action by regulatory and regulated bodies who define their educational objectives along juridical lines. However, feedback also offers a privileged space for speaking back to medical authority from an exteriorized location. "Affect is not a personal feeling, nor is it a characteristic: it is an effectuation of a power of the pack that throws the self into upheaval and makes it reel" (Deleuze & Guattari, 1987, 240). Words such as "betweeness", "towardness" and "awayness" and "aboutness" are used by Ahmed (2004) and Massumi (2002) in an attempt to fill an expressive void while acknowledging the movement that occurs in and between events, experiences, and bodies. Words can only approximate the relational and energetic nature of what goes on in such exchanges and I wonder about the limits of communication and the possibilities of translating what is knowable through emotion and affect except through the body. For SPs a line of flight occurs in the speaking back to medical authority through affective engagements that exceed words chosen to describe the work of embodying suffering. "Affect transpierces the body like arrows, they are weapons of war that derterritorialize" (Deleuze & Guattari, 1987, p. 356).

3.8   Towards a Nomadic Ethics: "So that is how you survive?"

At stake in this discussion of affect and emotion is the possibility of a practical ethics that revalues failure and in which contingency can be taken into account. "One has to think the unthinkable and imagine the unimaginable. In other words one has to contemplate "the unedifying spectacle of one's failings or shortcomings" (Braidotti, 2006, p.201). As

Braidotti suggests, "the ethical life is not given: it is a project...the conditions which allow for this must be immanent and depend on external circumstances and therefore on others" (Braidotti, 2006, p. 201).

Ethics as an embodied practice, "includes the acknowledgement of and compassion for pain, as well as the activity of working through it" (Braidotti, 2006, 267). For Doctor Smith this means suspending his ideas about who Mr. Skinner is and what he needs in order to make space for the unknown and the emergent. As filtered through Dr. Smith's expert clinical eye, Mr. Skinner's life is reduced to a series of needs - relief of pain, social supports, and access to resources such as the home care nurse - ironically disembodied; much like food that is eaten not for pleasure but solely for nutrients. It is hard to swallow. In conversation with the SP in the large group following the encounter, the SP identified his offence at the question about hockey at the end of the exchange. It wasn't asked out of genuine interest in his life or even as an attempt to get to know him but as part of an ongoing fact gathering activity to determine the patient's level of depression and/or competence for making decisions. It was transparent to all including Doctor Smith that he had reduced Mr. Skinner to an object and an agenda that needed to conform to his clinical needs. This occurred at a level between them that was "under verbal" – it was taking place in the invisible space both below and above their words and gestures. What seemed invisible was affectively alive and building-up like an electric charge in the space between them.

This is a risky space in which on the way to creating assemblages that are not subjectified, discomfort may be experienced as hierarchies give way to mutually nourishing relationships/assemblages. The SP and the doctor are engaged in a nomadic activity of following and listening to the "in between" which they both inhabit. This fertile space of possibility is not required to be filled with solutions but questions and problems as an ongoing creative engagement. As a nomadic activity which takes place in the transitions between potentially contradictory positions Mr. Skinner and Dr. Smith are a "body–machine", defined by Braidotti as "an embodied, affective and intelligent entity that captures, processes and transforms energies and forces" (Braidotti, 2006, p. 267). It is this engagement of force as a mutual undertaking that holds promise for incorporation of difference.

"Ethics as a practice is related to a play of complexity that encompasses all levels of one's multi layered subjectivity, binding the cognitive to the emotional, the intellectual to the affective and connecting them all to a socially embedded ethics of sustainability" (Braidotti, 2006, p.156). SP exchanges with medical trainees and practicing health professionals offer opportunities for ethical and aesthetic commitment to learning as a form of mutual metamorphosis and mutation. These opportunities become part of a sustainable ethical commitment through an obligation to surfacing privileged perspectives and their effects in the moment of exchange. This requires that spaces be made for thinking and behaving differently or for what Ahmed refers to as a space of wonder. For Ahmed, "The capacity for wonder is the space of opening up to the surprise of each combination; each body, which turns this way or that, impresses upon others, affecting what they can do. "Wonder keeps bodies and spaces open to the surprise of others" (2004 p. 183). For as Michael Hardt suggests, "We do not know in advance what a body can do, what a mind can think, - what affects they are capable of" (Hardt, 2007, p. x). Ahmed talks about wonder as a key affective space created when emotion cannot be translated into an outcome.

This space where outcomes are held back in order to keep open the possibility of discovery is the liminal edge of a pedagogy in which bodies actively engage in emotional and affective work. Such an approach acknowledges all of "our proximity to the crack" (Braidotti, 2006, p. 261), creating a space for discovery and the possible growth of an ethics through aesthetics. Such an ethics collectively acknowledges and works to move us beyond the notion of the individual as a container of emotion asking us to question the split between emotion and rationality. It is what Braidotti refers to as a nomadic ethics premised on subjectivity defined in terms of becoming. Such an ethics is situated and attached to our relationships and interactions with others or as Deleuze would suggest by way of Spinoza "our capacity to affect and be affected.

In the John Murrell play *Waiting for the Parade,* (1977), a community of women in small town Prairie Canada during World War II shares their life stories. My favourite line from the play is, "Oh so that is how you survive." It is spoken by a woman whose husband is missing in action in response to a story told by Marta, a daughter of German parents about her ostracism by the community. I always remember it as a statement of wonder and acknowledgement of mutual struggle that enacts a powerful and transformational witnessing. There is no solution to each of the character's suffering, no end point other than communal witnessing. Murrell suggests as much in an interview speaking about this play.

> In every action and every response that we have, if we develop memory as a strong organ, we can bring all of our past and all of the past of all of our people, virtually, forward with us into every instant of life. We can bring all of the wisdom, passion, and perception of

beauty that we've ever had. (John Murrell in 1994 interview, Canadian Theatre Encyclopedia).

3.9 Conclusion

Teaching is an embodied cultural and political undertaking that shapes and is shaped by emotion and affect. The ways in which emotion and affect are acknowledged and engaged in SP teaching work encourages us to follow expanded paths to understanding and making meaning out of day to day professional interactions.

In this chapter I have mapped emotion and affect as socio-cultural forces which are embedded in medical education practice and the implications for standardized patient teachers' embodied pedagogy. Offering an alternative nomadic ethics that acknowledges loss and failure as starting points I have put forward the suggestion that ethics is a practice of wonder and witnessing.

The following chapter provides a genealogy of medical simulation in which SPs and their role within this larger field of technology will be examined. The technological imaginary that constructs various medical simulation modalities will be explored, as well as the location of SPs and the absence/presence of emotion and affect within the field.

Notes

1. See MargaritShildrick, (2002). *Embodying the Monster: Encounters with the Vulnerable Self.* London, Thousand Oaks, New Delhi: Sage Publications. For a full genealogical feminist analysis of theories of the female body.

2. I am indebted to Jamie Lynn Magnusson for this distinction between hierarchical and nomadic assemblages and praxis.

3. War machines are integral to Deleuze and Guattari's nomodology and will be further explicated in chapter 6. They state "It is not enough to affirm that the war machine is external to an apparatus. It is necessary to reach the point of conceiving the war machine as itself a pure form of exteriority, whereas the State apparatus constitutes the form of interiority we habitually take as a model, or to which we are in the habit of thinking. (Deleuze & Guattari, 1987, p. 354).

4. I am capitalizing "State" following Deleuze and Guattari's example from *a thousand plateaus.* Their use of upper and lower case are themselves a comment on the relations between various organizations, institutions and ideas. Hence war machine and nomad are lower case along with royal science which places them in relation to each other and the State in different ways.

5. *Final Exit* is a book of recipes outlining different methods committing suicide.

Chapter 4 The Field of Medical Simulation: An Overview

The tradition of reproduction of the self from the reflections of the other - the relation between organism and machine has been a border war. The stakes in the border war have been the territories of production, reproduction, and imagination (Haraway, 1991, p. 150).

4.0 The Market Place

The hotel lobby is alive with activity as booths are assembled with full bodies laid out on tables, accompanying exchangeable latex body parts, and computer screens aglow with virtual games and the latest simulation applications all accompanied by the theme from Star Wars. Paramedics wander the hall bursting into seemingly spontaneous rescue procedures with mannequins on stretchers and assorted medical paraphernalia in action. A popcorn stand, a bean bag toss and other attractions are scattered throughout the mid-size hotel hall. This is a simulation symposium: a networking opportunity with industry and government and education representatives in attendance. The word of the day is inter-professionalism in the service of innovation and expansion of simulation technology in health care education. It is a carnival atmosphere – intentionally constructed to make the day fun, creative. As with all carnivals, the shiny surfaces and games serve to seduce on the one hand and divert attention from the real business of selling on the other.

Medical simulation is an industry with millions of dollars at stake. Links between investment in innovation of new hardware and software, through collaboration between industry, government and education are essential for its sustainability. In this assemblage communication and humanity are used as practical (skill acquisition) and moral (reduction of suffering through practice) tropes supporting the necessity of commercial expansion. Live patients, where represented in video displays or on posters as part of research, are peripheral to the main business of high tech happenings and theatrical display. It would seem there is little money to be made in talk between live people unmediated by high technology. This is a simple story with complicated implications for resource allocation, legitimacy and ownership of colonizing methodologies. Notions of embodiment, affect and emotion are being shaped and sold in packages underpinned by modernist assumptions that dichotomize and exclude. Medical simulation is a multi-million dollar education industry in which human relations, although part of the equation, are subordinated to overarching objectives for creating and perfecting systems in which interaction needs to be controlled and accounted for as part of those systems. Where there is force however there is resistance and productive possibilities. This is also part of the continuing story.

4.1   Introduction

This chapter provides a genealogy of the field of medical simulation and the place of human simulation and the work of standardized patients within it. How did I get here? As a trained actor steeped in the humanities, what is the relationship between the mechanical, virtual and plastic world of medical simulation and the living breathing world I inhabit as a SP scholar and teacher? I will provide an overview of different modalities within the field of medical simulation and some of the socio- historical conditions which have provided possible impetus to their development. As well I will discuss the implications for human simulation located within the field and the absent presence of emotion and affect.

4.2 Background

Simulation broadly conceived covers a range of concepts and activities which are socio culturally derived. In other words the field and meanings within it are part of a dynamic process of discursive practices and materialities, fluctuating according to particular contexts and applications. At its broadest, simulation refers to the representation or reproduction of something real through imitation. In medical education specifically it refers to: physical objects that can be substituted for the real thing (mannequins, part task trainers), activities related to representing a process or skill (resuscitation, suturing), as well as complex environments that reproduce technical, and environmental conditions (laparoscopic and haptic trainers, virtual worlds and operating room environments).

Technological expansion within medical simulation has been accompanied by a plethora of terminology, much of it confounding. Of particular interest to me are the assumptions embedded in the usage of different terms and the political work it entails. In some instances common terms are used to describe different activities and concepts while in others, different names describe the same concepts. The term "medical simulation" is a catch all signifier that positions SPs as a "modality" within its borders. The term "modality" has a particular meaning within medicine as a "prescribed treatment or procedure". "Living simulators" or SPs are positioned very particularly within a web of educational treatments. Power to include as well as exclude possible actions, positions of authority, and access to resources is embedded in the ways we describe objects and activities, making language and its effects inherently political. How is emotion transformed through simulation technology and how do various modalities imagine human bodies, emotion and affect within medical education training?

4.3 Genealogy of Medical Simulation

Simulation in this examination is understood to be a technique or application, while technology is the means for carrying it out. Simulation in medical education today and the work of standardized patients are shaped by medicine's focus on professionalism in the latter part of the 20th century an increased societal demand, globally, for accountability, and a resulting rationale that informs medical education reform. A medical professionalism internally focused on defending its privilege of self-regulation in the face of increasing societal dissatisfaction has redefined itself along the lines of competencies and roles. "For instance, to meet minimum requirements to practice medicine in Canada, physicians need to demonstrate over two hundred profession specific and team based competencies as mandated in the Royal College of Physicians and Surgeons of Canada (RCPSC) CanMEDS competency framework and the Canadian Patient Safety Institutes 2008 safety framework" (Reeves, 2009, p. 452). Competency as a core construct within professional training has produced a recognized need for pedagogical techniques and tools amenable to practice, observation and measurement of skills, to which simulation methodologies are ideally suited.

The history of "medical simulation", (mannequins, part task trainers etc.) and human simulation have grown in parallel but from different lineage. Medical simulation has roots in the fields of aeronautics, military and industrial design (Bradley, 2006; Rosen, 2009), while the arts and humanities inform the emergence of human simulation within medical education. Both the living and non living modalities meet medical profession's need for observable skills acquisition through practice. Despite the similar applications within medical education, there is a startling gap pedagogically and aesthetically between simulation practitioners, especially between those engaged in human simulation and those working with mechanized, computer and virtual technological approaches. Nevertheless, despite the gap, the emphasis on materials and what they can be made to do informs a notion of standardized patients and what they can be made to perform as malleable and passive material. There is epistemological affinity between "live" and "not live" modes of simulation, premised on the value of experiential learning. However the two approaches originate from within different paradigms and their trajectories although apparently similar, reflect distinctive notions of the relationships between embodiment as well as learning about and from bodies.

Rather than dichotomize the technological and the human which only further reifies a Cartesian split between reason and emotion, mind and body, it is more helpful for me to ask the question: How do technologies and humans interact to create different possibilities for experience of emotion and its expression in particular contexts? I am interested in embodied performative relationships between emotion and technology with the understanding that: "Learners' can interact *with* technology, *through* technology, and *within* a technological context, but on each occasion our meaning making abilities and embodied lives are central" (Zembylas, 2005, 193-4). What follows is an overview of the socio cultural backdrop within which both forms of simulation activities take place.

4.3.1 From Military to Medicine

> Modern states, multinational corporations, military power, welfare state apparatuses, satellite systems, political processes, fabrication of our imaginations, labour-control systems, medical constructions of our bodies, commercial pornography, the international division of labour, and religious evangelism depend intimately upon electronics. Micro-electronics is the technical basis of simulacra; that is, of copies without originals (Haraway, 1991, p.165).

Advances in the aeronautics industry beginning with Edwin Link the inventor of the first blue box flight trainer in the 1930's and the subsequent adoption of simulation technologies by industry, government and military, has provided the ground and inspiration for medical simulation. Essential antecedents to this growth were innovations in flight simulation, resuscitation, technology, and plastics. "Computers facilitated the mathematical description of human physiology and pharmacology, world wide communication, and the design of virtual worlds" (Smith, 2000, cited in Rosen 2008, p.157).

In the U.S, large scale investment by federal regulators, the Department of National Defence, and business, including the National Aeronautics and Space Administration (NASA) and nuclear power industry have made simulation a potent legitimizing activity. "The military was a major impetus in the transfer of modeling and simulation technology to medicine" (Loftin, 2002, p.16). The foundations for modern day medical simulation have been laid over the last twenty to thirty years partly in response to levels of inexperience of medical personnel in treating the type of casualties found in the field during the Gulf War.

4.3.1.2 Military Theatre

More recently as "America's embedment in the Middle East has become increasingly entrenched, complicated and violent, the Armed Forces are looking to theatre and performance for new counterinsurgency strategies to keep apace with the shifting specificities of the present war"[1] (Magelssen, 2009, p. 47). The National Training Centre has created vast simulations of war environments for preparation of combatants going over to Iraq and Afghanistan. Termed, "Theatre Immersions" the simulations involve the creation of entire villages, "living breathing environments complete with residential, governments retail, and worship districts- bustling with costumed inhabitants" (Magelssen, 2009, p. 48). Likened by one trainer to "improvised Shakespearean plays", the scenario writers are playwrights, the villagers, actors; and the staff who make sure everything is pulled off correctly the stage managers" (Magelssen, 2009, p. 52). The largest of these environments termed "The Sandbox" is described as "a virtual space of play and experimentation, and a mirror reproduction of the real Iraq" (Magelssen, 2009, p.48). The goal of the two week exercise is for the soldiers to "learn to live and work sensitively with Iraqi civilians, to mediate in sectarian and ethnic conflict, and to gain trust, all the while trying not to produce more insurgents by making mistakes. As reported in 2006 in a *New York Times* article, (Filkins& Burns 2006 as cited in Magelssen, p. 49). "With actors and stuntmen on loan from Hollywood, American Generals have recast the training ground of Fort Irwin so effectively as a simulation of conditions in Iraq and Afghanistan […] that some soldiers have left with battle fatigue and others have had their deployment to war zones cancelled. In at least one case, a soldier's career was ended for unnecessarily 'killing civilians" (Magelssen, 2009, p. 49).

This report echoes the article by the Los Angeles Times in 1964 regarding the breach of professional boundary through the use of "actors" in medical school settings, however there is not the same derogatory gendered overtone.

Similar to human simulation in medical education, there is a complex and shifting commitment to "reality" at play. The Iraqi actors, who are for this exercise "Arabic speaking Iraqi expatriates from Detroit, San Diego and other cities", are positioned ambiguously. "Operating tactically in another's space, they stage Iraq and portray their countrymen for Americans, with agendas sometimes similar to those of the American and sometimes all their own" (Magelssen, 2009, p.50). On a much smaller scale people portraying patients for medical professionals are similarly in another's space enacting stories that although not necessarily their own may carry personal meaning that many leak into the interactions in which they participate. Likewise, there are real physical, mental and emotional effects experienced by SPs following the portrayal of certain roles (McNaughton 1999). There is also commitment articulated by the actors both in the war simulation and SPs in medical settings to their altruistic contribution to the larger field in which they are working. In the war simulation one of the actors expressed appreciation for the difference she is making saving lives. "It pleases her to know she's doing good, while another sees it as teaching the troops how to avoid error" (Magelssen, 2009, p. 61). SPs have also stated that they are committed to the work despite low pay because they feel they are contributing to medicine and bettering patient care through their work (McNaughton, 1999).

A pressing question voiced by those involved in war theatre immersions is: Are the American soldiers in training also actors? This is also a concern voiced within medical education settings. Are we turning our doctors into "acting doctors" performing empathy for patients? (Hanna & Fins, 2006). This question hints at the larger issue of authenticity and acting which is at the heart of many of the debates within human simulation. What is the relationship between imagination and the reproduction of roles such as soldier and doctor? As suggested by Haraway in the opening quote: "The tradition of reproduction of the self from the reflections of the other - the relation between organism and machine has been a border war (1991, p. 150). In medical simulation one such border is between the mannequin technologies that stand in for the real patient and the professionalizing doctors who are reproducing professional selves through relationships with these machines and through further creation of the technology that reinscribes their professional identity.

With respect to the environments in which the simulations are taking place, there is a commonality between a militarized efficiency of medical performance examinations – OSCEs - that require logistical coordination and specific timing of events and movement of bodies and the complex algorithms that inform military manoeuvres, the more so for "games" that require the apparently naturalistic unfolding of events. There is nothing naturalistic about the organization or intent of a multi station OSCE. However the activity that takes place behind each exam room door is meant to represent the reality of a patient/doctor encounter with attending props, makeup and costume.

4.3.2 Patient Safety and Medical Error Reduction

Concerns about medical error, patient safety and human factors are the cornerstones for the growth of investment in medical simulation today driven by increasingly sophisticated technologies. Beginning with the aeronautics industry, safety enhancement and error reduction have been key justifications for the development and investment in medical simulation technology. "What the aeronautics industry, military and nuclear power industry have in common is that for each of them, training or systems testing in the "real" world would be too costly or too dangerous to undertake" (Bradley 2006, p. 255). Economic factors are always a central concern for investment in and use of simulation. Humans do not escape this net any more than machines do and are evaluated on their value according to feasibility, sustainability and reliability of outcome. Another event within medicine which advanced a rationale for an institutional approach and agenda on patient safety was the widely respected publication of two seminal articles; *To Err is Human* (Kohn, 2000), and, *An Organization with a Memory* (Department of Health, 2000). *To Err is Human* is cited as being referenced over one million, three hundred thousand times on a Google search of the book. Both of these publications provide a systematic overview and list of recommendations that justify the value of increased activity in medical simulation market. There are currently national organizations and conferences dedicated to patient safety and medical error reduction providing a societal voice in the call for medical simulation to be supported provincially (NECSTL)[2] ,internationally (SSIH)[3] and professionally.[4]

Interest in "human factors" and reduction of error has led to a focus on systems approaches to the interface between machine and human activity.

It was found as early as 1979 that; "Human factors were implicated as contributory in most air safety problems" (Rosen 2008, p. 158). This is a growing field of engineering within medicine that is committed to the design and redesign of user friendly tools that will reduce human error and includes among others: operating room checklists, I.V. equipment and e-medical records. Of interest for this discussion is the focus on preventing human error as if it were a simple matter of knowledge and rational choice. It does not take into account that errors are inevitable. There is no system that will eradicate "human" factors from human interaction and so such focus rationalizes investment of further time not in the human elements of medicine, but, rather ironically, constructs all human interaction as problematic and needing to be managed by an objective system of control.

4.4   Medical Simulation

The use of inanimate models in medical practice is traceable by some accounts back to the 15th century and perhaps even earlier. Paracelsus (1493-1541), an alchemist and physician was said to have attempted the resuscitation of a corpse using bellows, a trick he perhaps picked up from some Arabic medical writings" (Harris, 1992, p. 25). "The first recorded use of a medical simulator for training is that of a manikin created in the 17th Century by a DrGregoire of Paris (Buck, 1991, p. 7). He used a pelvis with skin stretched across it to simulate an abdomen, and with the help of a dead foetus he taught about assisted and complicated deliveries to midwives. "Physical models of anatomy and disease were constructed long before the advent of modern plastic and computers" (Rosen, 2008, p. 157).[5]

Engagement of materials dead and living (human and animal) in order to learn through practice also reminds us of the long history of cadaver use and grave robbing that accompanied early adoption of the practice of anatomy dissection (Harris, 1992). Practice with animated and inanimate materials in the name of science and for the benefit of patients is connected morally and affectively to the idea and actuality of simulation activities, placing such learning within a socio cultural and political landscape as well as medical.

4.4.1 Fidelity

Fidelity is a key value concept within medical simulation that threads through discussions of the merit and shortcomings of different modalities. A contentious term within the simulation field, fidelity can be employed to mean different things in different contexts, with important implications for access to resources. As a concept it attends to notions of realism as a result of the model itself, (the feel of the skin, facial expression, etc.), to the realism of environment and, also, to the quality of the experience for the learner. The latter concern invites us to look beyond traditional instrumentalist notions of technology as neutral to one in which technology can be seen to "generate new forms of emotional experience and identity formation" (Zembylas, 2005, p. 193). For example low fidelity describes the rudimentary nature of models such as a paper cup with two straws inserted at different angles to practice kidney stone removal. Such a tool for practicing kidney stone removal was developed by Matsumotto and colleagues (2002) who successfully showed effectiveness for skills acquisition using inexpensive low fidelity models. (Matsumotto, Hamstra, Radomski, Cusimano, p.1244). High fidelity describes either equipment such as mannequins who look and respond physically in a realistic manner to clinical examinations and procedures or haptic trainers that simulate what a procedure would feel like to the clinician (Issenberg, 2005). It also describes whole environments such as an operating room set up for surgery with all the attending sounds and suite of machines that need to be coordinated and managed as well as a responding mannequin. So a team of surgeon, nurses, anaesthetist can practice together as they would during an actual operation.

SPs are referred to as both high and low fidelity by those in medical simulation. SPs are considered high fidelity when they contribute to the emotional and affective realism of a clinical situation or when their bodies can be used for practicing different non invasive procedures, such as injuries for mocked up wound dressings or appendicitis for physical exam practice. It has been suggested that the "experience of interacting with an actual living person makes them "more real" and better suited for helping students to develop (and instructors to assess) clinical skills, especially communication skills" (Taylor, 2011, p. 137). This advantage extends to the idea that they are not the "real thing" and therefore it is assumed cannot be hurt. "Indeed, some in the SP field group human actors (the so-called "wetware") together with computer simulators, virtual reality devices, and high-tech "realistic" computerized mannequins" (Taylor, 2011, p. 137). They are also sometimes considered low fidelity because as living people SPs are unable to fake certain clinical findings or be involved in invasive procedures. Therefore, where a label of low fidelity might be positive when referring to inert materials adapted for innovative and cost effective use as in the Matsumotto study, it is a negative when attached to living bodies who are unable to enact more complex physical findings or take part in invasive clinical procedures.

4.4.2 Medical Simulation Modalities

4.4.2.1 Part Task Trainers

The development of Resusci-Annie in 1960 by a Norwegian toy manufacturer, AsmundLaerdal, working with anaesthetists, proved a crucial step in the development of medical simulation as a field of its own. She was originally designed for mouth to mouth breathing. "Her face was based on the death mask of the *Girl from the River Seine,* a famous French drowning victim. Laerdal wanted to encourage the practice of rescue techniques by designing a sympathetic simulated victim" (Rosen, 2008, p. 160). The development of Resusci-Annie revolutionized "resuscitation training and became the prototype for part task trainers in medical education. Part task trainers are inanimate bench models or box-trainers made from synthetic materials to replicate a specific anatomical region of the body. The models represent only part of the real thing and will often comprise a limb or body part or structure...[with] some provid[ing] feedback (visual, auditory or printed) to the learner on the quality of their performance) e.g., simple clicking to represent adequate depth of chest compression in cardiopulmonary resuscitation (Bradley, 2006, p. 257-8). Within a few years Annie was joined by a "Harvey" a full body part task trainer. Developed at the University of Miami for focused practice with cardiac diagnosis and exam, Harvey was the first cardiology patient simulator programmed to simulate twenty seven different cardiac conditions.

4.5 A Brief History of Mannequins

4.5.1 Full Body Mannequins

The first full body simulator was constructed for the department of anaesthesia at the University of Southern California, San Diego, at the same time (1964) and in the same institution as Howard Barrows was attempting to introduce simulated patients. Not to be confused with full body *part tasktrainers*, the importance of these full body models was the increased range of systems that could be engaged. Rosen (2008) tells us that "SIM" "was produced by engineer Stephen Abramson, physician Judson Denson, and Aerojet General Corporation. The financial stimulus for development was the search for peacetime applications of Aerojet in light of diminished military spending (Cooper, 2004, p. 12). "Sim 1's facial features included blinking eyes, pupils that could change size, and an opening jaw" (Cooper, 2004, p. 12). His chest moved as if breathing and he had a heart beat that was synchronized with carotid and temporal pulse and associated with blood pressure. "The mannequin demonstrated a response to a handful of drugs and allowed performance of basic airway management" (Rosen, 2008, p. 161). Although it was a technological wonder the "Sim One" failed to achieve acceptance at this time. Both the cost of the technology and the lack of pedagogical method meant that it would not be until the 1980's before this modality really caught on.

At this time two groups, one at Stanford and the other at University of Florida, both from within anaesthesia, partnered with aeronautical manufacturing companies to develop, within two years of each other, sophisticated full body simulators. The philosophy and mission of the two groups were distinct and different. The Stanford team was focused on team performance during critical incidents patterning their training program after crew resource management (CRM) training from within flight simulation. The Florida group used their simulator to introduce their residents to anaesthesia techniques, common errors and machine failures. "The prototypes developed in California and Florida became commercial products during the 1990's" (Rosen, 2008, p. 161).

Full body simulators with a narrower focus also became more prevalent in the 1990's. As well as "Harvey" the full body cardiology simulator, the Gaumard Scientific Company developed a birthing simulator that included a new born mannequin capable of central and peripheral cyanosis" (Rosen, 2008, p. 162). These task specific simulators came to be known as "human patient simulators" further confounding understanding about the differences between human, live, and patient simulation as terms with any coherence. "Human patient simulation" infiltrated undergraduate medical education as an effective method to teach introduction to physical diagnosis and in some instances replacing animal exercises" (Rosen, 2008, p. 162). Health professions such as nursing have also developed fully equipped simulation centres with requisite full ward set ups and storage area for various limbs, sim babies, birthing mothers.

Commercial developments and competition between companies marketing the mannequin technology came to dominate the medical simulation field in the 1990's and to a large extent the educational agenda. Companies such as CAE http://www.cae.com/en/about.cae), (a descendent of the original Link Aeronautical Corporation that produced the pioneering "Link Trainer"), licensed models from Stanford's Comprehensive Anaesthesia Simulation Environment (CASE) technology and Harvard's Anaesthesia Simulation Centre (ASC) for commercialization. CAE is now in partnership with medical simulation centres within health professional institutions all over the world. The institutions receive state of the art simulation equipment for their students to train on and in exchange CAE acquire legitimacy through their connection with an academic institution for future marketing and business.

4.6   Social and Ethical Concerns

Technological developments take place in conjunction with and are shaped by social political and cultural influences. The tensions that arise as a result of costs and competition in the medical simulation field echo the ethically charged relationships in play between pharmaceutical companies and physicians. The "Boys with Toys" as the high tech simulation promoters have been dubbed are effectively positioned to direct heath professional educational curriculum from their academic capitalist commercially competitive perch. A large professional association, the Society for Simulation in Healthcare (SSIH) have successfully launched a movement to accredit simulation centres, one factor of which will be the amount and kind of simulation equipment being used (Issenberg, 2006, p. 203). The international Association for Standardized Patient Educators (ASPE) who are now firmly connected with SSIH are included in the accreditation net. However, it is a different situation for SP programs as they are designed in direct response to educational need rather than technological advantage. Human bodies don't receive technological improvements, and standards of operation relevant for machines do not necessarily fit humans. Accreditation is a controversial topic for human simulation programs and rightly so as it is a discourse in which power accrues through surveillance and normalization technologies eventually influencing access to resources, authority to make decisions and definitions of legitimate activity. Some fear that the smaller and mostly female human simulation field are being colonized by a growing industrial commercial "State apparatus."

9/11 was a critical moment in the advancement of high fidelity, high technical simulation perpetuating and justifying the tightening bonds between medical training and the military industrial complex. The U.S. government provided funding for the development of sophisticated simulation equipment making it available through grants to medical and military simulation centres no matter how small or inexperienced. A surge in the growth of simulation centers attached to academic centres ensued. There are over fifty-five in Ontario alone and this number is growing with every hospital rationalizing a need for high tech equipment for training purposes. According to one Director of an internationally renowned Medical Simulation Centre, "Millions of dollars of simulation equipment granted to Centres have never made it out of the boxes in which it was delivered". In many simulation centers there are few staff experienced in setting up or running the equipment let alone have the knowledge or time to train in how it might be educationally integrated. The growing commercialization and corporatization of medical professional training promoted by such advances is being met with critical attention. Academic capitalism is at work, as educational and pedagogical improvement has been called for by the leaders within the field in order to create a scholarly rationale for the expense and proliferation of all the different types of medical simulation technology. Such moves are "inescapably implicated in the flows of neo-colonialism, corporate capitalism, and other contemporary declensions of the mercantile and totalitarian hubris" (O'Roley, 2003, p. 68).

"Actors" or "confederates" are essential to mannequin based simulation but are rarely included in articles about this modality. They are living people who interact with the mannequin and the learner while in a role in order to assist both the technical and non technical aspects of the simulation. They are often technicians who are knowledgeable about the capabilities and limitations of the mannequin model and are present often first and foremost to make sure the "user" (student) doesn't break the equipment and while there also "acts as" the other health professional to take directions and assist in medical interventions. The only mention I have seen is reference in a published abstract for a workshop describing its objectives as follows, "This immersive workshop will demonstrate an effective use of confederate actors with the human patient simulator to help convey best practices of teaching advanced cardiac life support to health care providers" (http://www.hpsn.com/event/hpsn-annual-2012/67/#tab_workshopsandcourses). They are most often non clinicians who are trained in a specific simulation modality (i.e., Harvey) with knowledge of particular educational objectives (Demaria, et.al. 2010). In this way they are like SPs. There is very little known about their experience in these settings. We do know that students can be emotionally affected by the experience of having a mannequin die or go into distress and so attention has been increasingly directed toward training the "actor" also tellingly called a "confederate" in briefing and debriefing techniques in order to both prepare learners for the experience as well as to debrief around any negative effects. As the term "confederate" suggests there are complex power alignments similar to those for SPs in teaching settings. With whom are the technicians conspiring?

It is ironic that this activity in this setting is referred to as "acting" while SP educators engaged in portraying patient stories have gone to great lengths to develop terminology that effectively distances them from this term despite it describing an essential aspect of their activity. Nowhere in the official website for live simulation, the Association of Standardized Patient Educators (ASPE) will the term actor appear. As the popularity of model based simulation including part task trainers grows there are possibilities created for different kinds of interactions and relationships: between learners, teachers and learners, third party interlocutors and finally between learner and machine. Presently the focus is on developing these different relationships as skills that can be practiced with little attention to the production and reproduction of ideas and professional values related to patient care.

4.7 Virtual and computer based systems

Virtual reality refers to the re-creation of environments or objects as a complex computer generated image: haptic systems refer to those replicating the kinaesthetic and tactile perception (Bradley, 2006). Computer technologies have been increasingly incorporated into mannequin and model based simulation in order to create more realistic and "immersive" simulation environments. Concern with improving the realism of technology and potential fidelity of experience, suggests the importance of affect and its relationship to the simulated body and its responses. However it also signals the centrality of the affective experience of the clinician learner as a method of "improving" empathy. O'Riley asks, "Is virtual learning yet another form of colonization, the next frontier? Colonizing and domesticating technology discourses by organizing so-called systems of knowledge organizes and controls people"

(2003, p. 68). We find ourselves in the State apparatus as part of a control society as imagined by Deleuze and Guattari.

The first virtual reality system known as Sensorama was created by Morton Helig between 1956 and 1961 at which time it was released as a commercial product. "The apparatus projected images, vibration, sound, smell and wind to deliver five different immersive experiences" (Rosen, 1020, p. 162). Second Life, a virtual world, was initiated in 2003. In a few short years this application has registered almost ten million accounts with many Universities purchasing real estate or "islands" in order to enhance distance learning (Ellaway, 2008).

Virtual medical simulation first appeared in 2007 in the community known as *Ann Meyers Medical Center* (Mesko, 2007). Because avatars of users from around the world can interact online it has been thought that this application would serve to provide medicine a global platform. "Computer constructs are more easily assessed, more sanitized, and less troublesome than messy, imperfect, unpredictable physical bodies" (O'Riley, 2003, p. 110). However the uptake within many medical schools has been less than hoped for either as a result of expense or lack of pedagogy to meaningfully engage learning at a level worth the expense. As one Director of a simulation program at a Canadian Medical School remarked; "There are two issues, [one is that] Second Life, in and of itself, has actually no purpose whatsoever. The whole point of it is that you bring that purpose into it and build it into the environment. The second is that it lacks the subtleties that you need for proper simulation. It's rubbish for any kind of procedural skill because it's like wearing huge snow mitts. You can't manipulate anything." Remarking on the realism of VR in semiotic terms this Director identified the work of JorisDormans (2008) who writes about different kinds of realism in gaming simulation. She states:

> Iconic are like for like. Indexical are similar but not really the same. Symbolic are just representing but quite different. So, for instance, in virtual patient activity, I'm very active in developing virtual patient technologies and virtual patient content and the pedagogy of these virtual patients. But effectively, in a virtual patient you click on stuff or you type stuff and that's not the same as using your voice or an in-body reaction with the patient. So, there is a very symbolic nature to virtual patients, whereas the mannequin, when you palpate or you do a lot of the activities, they are exactly the same as you do. There's nuance that you have to adapt around a real human being but they're pretty much the same. So, within a simulation environment there is a real challenge over the iconic, symbolic relationship, and certainly in a virtual world like Second Life, although the social dimensions are very iconic pretty much everything else is very symbolic, or at most, indexical. It looks like it's real but you can't interact in a real way. So, our update of the [University's] islands has actually been pretty low and I think appropriately low because, although we developed it from R&D and a curiosity point of view, we have yet to find any significant use for it.[6]

In other words VR's lack of reception may result from a mismatch related to expectations that it provides another variation of a mannequin or live interaction, when this is not the case. The "user" has to leave this reality to learn in another less real reality which in the end does not provide an actual experience of skills transfer. Despite its lukewarm reception formally there is presently a proliferation of commercial virtual reality environments taken up by medical education with some laboratories adding the sense of touch through haptics. VR co-opts temporal and geographical metaphors. Students are "users". (like drug or game addicts)? Activities take place on an island that one arrives at and leaves from at scheduled times. It is a modality in search of a compelling pitch.

4.8 Human Cadaver and Animal Models

Cadavers and animals (anaesthetized and dead) are considered a sub-category of part-task training and are used in a variety of medical and surgical specialties. According to the medical education literature a major use of cadaver and animal models seems to be to test the transferability of skills learned after training with other forms of simulation (e.g., Friedman, 2008), especially when transfer performance on patients is perceived as unethical or unnecessary. The use of cadaver and animal models in medical training is a difficult ethical topic that intersects with investigations of emotion as a site of critical learning. What kind of communication and critical judgement can be promoted in the context of such learning? Can ideas about power relations, professional and human privilege, and science be interrupted through embodied learning and made visible as critical praxis? A critical approach to engaging living and dead organic and plastic materials as technologies for learning recognizes the multi-dimensional relationship between emotion and reason. It also broadens our perspectives beyond the human regarding ethics, responsibility and practice in the pursuit of knowledge. There is no "us" and "them" with respect to life forms. Even technologically we are increasingly connected to and extended through techniques that challenge such simplistic divisions. Interrupting taken for granted truths about matter in its different forms engages learners in thinking about their embodied cognitive and affective investments in relationships.

4.9 Hybrid Simulation

More recently designing simulated body parts to attach to live people in what is called "hybrid simulation" is an increasingly popular means of expanding medical simulation teaching and assessment. Roger Kneebone and colleagues (2006) developed the concept of hybrid simulation whereby a standardized patient is combined with an inanimate simulator and/or other pieces of medical equipment. Wounds in need of suturing, penises in need of catheterization are attached to people who add an affective dimension to the procedure taking place. Feedback in this instance refers to sharing information with the leaner about not only the skill involved in the technical procedure but the "patient/model's" experience. An SP becomes cybernetic organism; "a creature of social reality as well as a creature of fiction" (Haraway, 1991, p. 469), with relationships structuring and structured by social reality beyond their own flesh.

We are in liminal territory here as living beings cross into a theatre of props and prostheses, while medical technology plays with ideas of fidelity and authenticity. Late twentieth century machines have made thoroughly ambiguous the difference between natural and artificial, mind and body, self-developing and externally designed, and many other distinctions that used to apply to organisms and machines" (Haraway, 1991, p.152). Increasingly our mentalities extend beyond our fleshy borders into devices which hold, store, define, produce… emotional meanings and experiences. As suggested by Haraway this is neither good nor bad but constitutive of new relationships that interrupt notions of real and fake in favour of the productive possibilities of simulacra: copies that come to stand in for no longer existing originals.

4.10 Human Simulation: Fleshy Mannequins

In parallel with the "use" of animals and cadavers as learning technologies, what sets human simulation apart from the mechanical medical simulation modalities is the essential place of ethics as a practice when students and teachers are in contact with corporeal matter. In the case of SPs, suffering can be caused to those hired to teach about the amelioration of suffering in ways that do not occur with mannequins or virtual characters (McNaughton, 1999). This further dimension is explicitly made visible and felt either as a presence (causing pain) or an absence (not acknowledging the pain caused). Janelle Taylor (2011) in her ethnographic study exploring SPs ideas about realism with respect to their simulation activities suggests that, "SP performances necessarily raise the same difficult, important, fundamentally ethical questions that are always involved in learning from and on human beings who are capable of suffering, and who need and deserve recognition and respect as well as care" (Taylor, 2011, p. 135). SPs can be and are occasionally hurt in their interactions in educational settings. This can occur physically, emotionally or both as well as socially. She states, "Another of the ethically awkward aspects of SP performances, is that although they are intended to protect "actual patients" from risk and suffering, they cannot avoid imposing a certain degree of risk and suffering on other people: the SPs themselves" (Taylor, 2011, p. 150). In terms of an absence of care Taylor points out it is ironic that some of the SPs she interviewed, portrayed patients who had greater access to healthcare and social resources than the SP playing the part. The ethics of engaging SPs in medical simulation activities asks medical educators to 'recognize, understand and engage the social and economic realities surrounding the work, the lives, and the health of SPs and "actual patients" alike" (Taylor, 2011, p.151).

The conception of physicians' activities as performative and illness as an art form to be constructed through a medical gaze sets a very different course for human simulation from that of medical simulation. As such: "The representation of medical signs and symptoms in literature or theatre can be imagined as precursors of non-technical simulation" (Rosen, 2008, p. 157). I will explore the special considerations that shape human simulation in the next chapter.

Interestingly, in an early reference to live simulation it is conceived in negative terms as a form of deception such as here defined by Robert South in 1697,

> […]for Distinction Sake, a Deceiving by Words, is commonly called a Lye, and a Deceiving by Actions, Gestures, or Behavior, is called Simulation (South, 1697, p.525)(http://en.wikipedia.org/wiki/Simulation).

The spectre of malingering or acting symptoms and signs in order to achieve secondary (personal) gain haunts the work of standardized patients. In other words SPs can use their role playing to gain proximity to practitioners in order to access help for their own suffering. Human simulation involves agency and encompasses positive and negative valences: enacting that which is "not present", as well as dissimulating – hiding that "which is present". Intent to deceive introduces power relations into human simulation in ways not possible with passive and pre-programmed models.

> Women it has been said are born actors. May not cunning and dissimulation so frequently found in the hysteric state be in some measure attributable to an innate tendency in this direction, evolved in the manner indicated? (Campbell, 1891 p. 54, as cited in Weber, 1911, p 29).

Once again I suggest that gender, women as actors and medical education form a potent combination that informs the possibilities and shape of SP work. Standardized patients are recognized as important to include within discussions occurring in the larger field of medical simulation, however there is a sense that what is on offer is a "high priced" fleshy version of the more adaptable, less messy, more accurate plastic and computerized mannequins. There is the possibility alluded to above that in fact SPs are just convincing liars – cunning (women) who intentionally deceive as do malingering patients for possible secondary gain. This thinking infiltrates the field itself influencing the criteria and processes for choosing new SPs. For example, it is an important consideration, one included in the SP program's formal documentation, that during the screening process for new SPs successful candidates have no hidden grudge against the medical profession for which they may use their potential doubly privileged closeness as knowing patient and teacher. There is an implied acknowledgement of the power to subvert that this location affords to SPs.

As I have discussed, in medical simulation SPs are considered "high fidelity", a term that has little currency or meaning for people enacting patient's stories. Fidelity is a notion born of scientists tinkering with tools in attempts to create "more" lifelike models or experiences. However, SPs are already more than life like, perhaps too much so for some. There is a perception that the possibility of displaced or leaky emotions attached to the person playing the patient needs to be managed. It is ironic that there is a drive for more "real" effects in plastic and digital media to capture what is in effect, intentionally erased in the human alternative through standardization. SPs are colonized through attempts by medical simulation practitioners to locate them along the spectrum of modalities to be known in order to be used, while also marginalized through a fundamental misunderstanding about the embodied nature of the work in which SPs engage.

Acting, although not agreed upon by all in the SP field as the core activity in which SPs engage, is the discipline with which the work has the most resonance with a rich and ongoing debate amongst SP educators about whether what SPs are doing can be called acting. There is a rich and exchange on the ASPE list serve which I have been granted permission to share here. In response to a question regarding training acting students as standardized patients, one respondent suggested that SPs do not act. "SP performance is not acting, unless it could be termed "method acting". That is the SP performs realistically and naturally as him or herself but with a different history. But I don't prefer them at all for their ability to "pretend" they are the patient. Real patients don't pretend and learners note immediately when the SP is not genuine, i.e. is acting. Another respondent with a background as a director and acting teacher responded: "Acting as a form of social performance does not refer only to what actors do on stage or film, what we might call aesthetic performance. Acting covers a much wider spectrum than that. ...We all act in various ways. Doctors act in their consultations. They do not pretend because no decent actor pretends for one second. Pretence is driven out early in actor training. There is more pretence in the world off the stage than on it. Actors *commit to behave* (italics in the original) as a situation, real, or imagined demands. Doctors act as the situation demands them to act, whether they feel like it or not. They act for real. This misunderstanding goes back a long way. Acting is in fact more about choice of behaviour. He goes onto suggest that there are at least five different modes of acting in SP work depending on the demands of the case. [7]

This is a complex issue. As we can see from this exchange there is a fine distinction between acting as it is understood in theatre studies and the role work in which SPs engage in live simulation which will be taken up further in the next chapter.

I see the work of SPs also more broadly in terms of a kind of performance that has the potential to act as a critical lens; something that Dwight Conquergood (1995) describes as a "commitment to praxis, to multiple ways of knowing that engage embodied experience with critical reflection…a caravan; a heterogeneous ensemble of ideas and methods on the move" (1995, p. 139-40). This discussion introduces elements for examination that are outside the present chapter and will be pursued in the next chapter.

4.11 Conclusion

In this chapter I have provided an overview of medical simulation and the various simulation modalities locating human simulation within the field. As well I have described the socio cultural influences that were an integral part of shaping the field and its trajectory within medical education. The role of bodies, emotion and affect were examined in their relation to the various techniques described.

As I have discussed in this chapter simulation as an activity is far from politically neutral. The message seems to be that where there are lives at stake whether through accidents in air, nuclear catastrophes or war, practice through simulation is required. Economically, the higher the stakes (mass casualties as opposed to single patient deaths) the more money is available for technological support of simulated practice.

The dominant discourses at work within medical simulation are tied to ideas about outcomes acquired in supported (safe) environments. It is a skills-based rationale which intersects in interesting ways with performance as understood within theatre theory and actor training. We can see Foucault's "anatamo-clinical" gaze at work in a medical profession's investment (professional and financial) in physiologically advanced simulation equipment (respiratory, cardiac) and the image of the corpse or unmoving body, not the live patient, as a pedagogical focus. In the *Birth of a Clinic* Foucault states: "that which hides and envelopes, the curtain of night over truth, is, paradoxically, life; and death on the contrary, opens to the light of day, the black coffer of the body" (Foucault, 1975, 166).

Bodies produced by various medical simulation technologies are inert products of diagnostic and physiological thinking. The body as a seat of motility and praxis is missing.

> The lived body constantly transforms itself and is in a state of perpetual flux. Skills are acquired through a process of "incorporation" – the process of bringing within the body that which occurs over time. It is also the process by which abilities sediment into unreflective fixed habits. They are enveloped within the

structure of the taken-for-granted body from which I *inhabit* the world (Leder, 1990, p.32).

Medical simulation is a disciplining technology productive of power which is dispersed multilaterally and "its exercise, though often invisible, permeates and indeed constitutes individual bodies within the social body" (Diedrich, 2007, p. 12).

Haraway suggests that there is no separation between the technological and the human.

> Technologies and scientific discourses can be partially understood as formalizations, i.e., as frozen moments, of the fluid social interactions constituting them, but they should also be viewed as instruments for enforcing meanings. The boundary is permeable between tool and myth, instrument and concept, historical systems of social relations and historical anatomies of possible bodies, including objects of knowledge. Indeed, myth and tool mutually constitute each other (Haraway, 1991, p. 164).

Such an understanding of the constitutive interplay between tool and social relations is especially apt in this discussion of medical simulation.

Emotion and affect are present in each of the simulation modalities just discussed even in their absence. To see rationality alone as the driving force is to suggest that "emotion and reason are separate entities which do not recognize that systems of reason are products of culturally and historically specific power relations" (Zembylas, 2005, p. 185). The work of standardized patients as mentioned at the beginning of the chapter, although implicated in these technological advances, did not emerge as a result of them. The rationales came afterwards to justify and colonize their involvement. In the next chapter I will explore different traditions that have influenced the emergence of a mostly female field of patient acting in medical education.

Notes

1. Please see Scott Magelssen, "Rehearsing the Warrior Ethos" TDR: The Drama Review, 53:1 (T201) Spring 2009. P. 47-71. Magelssen's study of "Theatre immersion and the simulation of Theatres of war describes similar issues of purpose, experience and fall out in terms strikingly parallel to human simulation in medical education settings

2. NESCTL was established in April 2007 through a grant from the Ontario Ministry of Health and Long Term Care (MOHLTC). It has recently been renamed "SIMone" It currently represents" over 50 simulation centres, seven standardized patient programs, more than 80 researchers and over 1,000 members." (Simulation Expo, program, Dec. 2010).

3. On the home page for The Society for Simulation and Healthcare is a notice "offering qualifying corporate members collaboration opportunities through the formation of the Corporate Council. This Corporate partnership will seek to promote the visibility and recognition of the science of simulation." http://www.ssih.org/SSIH/SSIH/Home/Default.aspx. Accessed on December 7, 2010. In this passage Simulations linked to ideas of "collaboration", and through this to innovation well as to science. Rhetorically, joining the "simulation" corporate club it is implied ensures networking opportunities (fiscal?) through collaboration and a scientific (legitimate) pursuit of simulation opportunities. Education as enterprise.

4. The Royal College's simulation task force has created the Accreditation Guide for Simulation Programs to develop educational standards for simulation centres in Canada. The Chair of the task force suggests; "One of the first steps in ensuring that education is being delivered uniformly is to accredit programs and make sure they educate at a high standard," "Then we can begin to better address our profession's continuing professional development, as well as our revalidation needs going forward."

5. For a full history of medical simulation please see K.R. Rosen (2008). Also, Bradley P. (2006). Both articles provide a full and interesting chronology of events in medical simulation in North America. My contribution in this section relies heavily on the research of these two researchers.

6. Taken from an interview that was part of a review of simulation for the Future of Medical Education in Canada (FMEC) Project for which ethics was granted.

7. . SP-trainer listserve, Tuesday December 8, 2009, 545pm.

Chapter 5 Human Simulation: a Mapping

5.0   Introduction

The following chapter maps a rhizomatic network that includes acting, emotion, hysteria, medicine, and the place of women patients and standardized patients in these arenas. It is intended as an alternative reading of the advent of standardized patients and women in medicine as educators and actors. Central to this exploration is a genealogy of hysteria and its alignment with human simulation as a specific kind of illness performance.[1] Mapping as a deconstructive process unfolds and expands discrete elements interacting at interstitial nodes of contact. In the case of SP performances of emotion within clinical contexts there are presumptions about the ideality of relationships between doctor and patient, and mimesis as it produces reality through representation.

My mapping then is an effort to deconstruct a linear and well worn path between two or more points; for example between mimesis and simulation, and between representation and reality. In attempting to follow a scent, instead of accepting and legitimizing what are already taken for 'truths', I am opening up different lines of thought and practice; unpacking and repacking experiences and the rules that shape them. While my reading involves deconstruction it also involves generative reconstructions – an anti genealogical movement if you will that makes new connections that unsettle and raise new questions about what has been taken for granted as stable.

I am introducing ideas and vocabulary from Deleuze and Guattari's alternative ontology of "becomings" as a way of interrupting notions of unitary, universal and stable identifications. For example, their "Body without Organs" (BwO) refers to a set of practices that attempts to dismantle the known and stable identity or self, rather than pursuing it. "The BwO is what remains when you take everything away. What you take away is precisely the phantasy, the significances, and subjectifications as a whole" (Deleuze & Guattari, 1987, p. 151). In refiguring the story of SPs in this way I am hoping to create space for new understandings and possibilities for the work in which we engage.

5.1   Duplicity/Representation

Although patients' throughout the history of medicine have been used educationally as models and instruments of learning, with the rise of interest in hysteria, never had such an articulated exploration of a disease process involved patients in so central a role. I argue that at the turn of the nineteenth century conditions exquisitely supported the relationship between theatre and medicine as duplicitous, by which I mean the patient's performance was a particular "doubling" or "re" presentation integral in the case of hysteria, to solidifying it within a positivist scientific enterprise of classification and nosology. I do not mean to suggest as do some (Thomas Szasz, 1996) that hysteria never existed as an illness, but rather that it became a conduit, through representation and performance, for the anxieties and ambitions during an age of social and political change. Hysteria was essentially a mercurial disorder that was rewritten from one age to the next, serving those who used it for various clinical but also political purposes. Defying reliable diagnostic categorization, the question beyond, *what* was being represented during patients' presentations is, on whose authorship and what science were the re-presentations based? "Biomedical sciences deploy and are themselves, the systems of representation" (Showalter, 1993, p. 290). They construct objects to be known and epistemological systems for particular ends. In this instance such systems were visible parts of the environment in which patients spent their lives and to which they were subjected everyday. "Charcot's clinic was organized primarily around the visual, the photographic, the theatrical and the spectacular" (Showalter, 1993, p. 309). As Gilman (1993) suggests; capturing signs and symptoms visually through photography legitimized hysteria as real, physical disease. Echoing Foucault he continues;

> To see a patient means to develop a technique for seeing, a technique that is "scientific": the patient in turn as the object of the medical gaze becomes part of the process of the creation and the ontological representation of the disease, a representation that is labeled hysteria (Gilman 1993, p. 353).

Also in this process, the gaze which attempts to create distance and objectivity in the name of diagnostic science is in fact frustrated by its own object which is essentially ephemeral.

Gilman, a scholar working in the area of hysteria, reinforces my own argument regarding standardized patients' privileged knowledge of a clinician's version of a patient case and impoverished relationship to any actual patient story. Gilman states, "For the patient knows how to be a patient only from the representations of the way physicians wish to see (and therefore to know) the patient as the vessel of a disease, not any disease but the disease of images – imagining hysteria" (Gilman, 1993, p. 359). Visual representation of disease entities was important in grounding a physician's authority in diagnosis and interpretation of signs and made possible an assemblage of technologies such as surveillance, observation, classification etc. Gilman contends that patients at Salpêtrière were surrounded by visual representations to which they had access. He states,

> On the rear wall of the ward, a permanent fixture of the room inhabited by the patients, is a chart recording the different phases of hypnosis, the stages that the patient is expected to pass through as she performs for her male audience. It is part of the world of the patient, a means through which to learn how to structure one's hysteria so as to make one an exemplary patient(1993, p. 349). [2]

The suggestion is that the hysterical patients weren't really suffering but faking symptoms for secondary gain. Although a great deal has been written about the variability and impossibility of hysterical symptomotology as performed by the patients, very little is written about what secondary gain may have been so enticing to have kept them engaged in such deception. This is a intricate power matrix within which the patient as willing subject is both "duped" into representations that are accepted as "appropriate" through visual signalling and also constrained to hide such a duplicitous relationship with their representation of signs in order to achieve the status as an "exemplary" patient.

SPs today are also part of such an assemblage of technologies, co-constructing cultural representations of illness along side healthcare professionals, albeit as paid co-conspirators not patients. They also know how to perform patients' stories by virtue of the representations that they are provided by physicians for ironically perhaps SPs are not usually allowed contact with the patients they represent. This separation is maintained out of respect for anonymity however it also suspiciously maintains physician privilege over the patient story in a way that echoes Charcot's orchestrated demonstrations.

Medicine's fascination with "capturing" and "labelling" the unpredictable and contingent aspects of clinical representations is still observable in cultural constructions of emotion in medicine by SPs. These are visibly manifest in categorizations of roles to be presented as real classifications by SPs. Whereas two of the stars of Charcot's presentations, Augustine and Blanch Wittman performed the three phases of a hysterical epileptic seizure[3] and other signs of illness, already decided upon as essentially female; patient cases performed by SPs are also gendered, and labelled by such names as the "harried housewife", "the anxious divorcee" suggesting a gendered causal relationship between affectivity and illness.

I argue that learning about and performing emotion and affect as if they are gendered physiological aspects of illness, reproduces and reifies the normative relationship already taken for granted by the medical profession and the public between irrationality and illness.

The following story is a glimpse inside the experience of an SP enacting a story of a depressed patient. I suggest that the lines between acting and illness are essentially blurred and are not easy to discern from a professional medical perspective. The ways in which SPs are engaged by the medical profession and engage with the emotional and affective elements of a story, I contend, echo their historical and hysterical sisters.

5.2   Heather's story

The following story was told to me by a standardized patient about her experience in role during an advanced psychotherapy teaching session for resident level trainees in which she portrayed a depressed patient. The responses are those of the SP in character. The SP is not depressed with a "sick and useless husband". She is not really angry at the psychiatrist for having more wealth and a job. However she is inside her body's response to the psychotherapy resident interviewer's acknowledgment of the gap between them. It is visceral and immediate.

"I started to turn in my chair toward her. I didn't mean to or want to. I had been not looking at her." "What does she know about what I am going through?" "Look at her over there." "She has money, she's a fucking psychiatrist." "I don't have any money - she has a job." "I don't have a job, just a sick and useless husband." What good is talking to her about my sick kid and my pathetic life?" And then she says…… "Oh. I don't get it. I know I don't really get what you are going through. How could I?" And I think…"it is like against everything that I am feeling I start to turn around toward her and I am shocked at what I see." "She is smaller, shrunken sort of, from what I remember at the beginning of the session and I swear her hair is standing on end like a little frightened bird." And I think,… "Oh my God that is how I am feeling." "I don't want to feel like that, I am sick of feeling like that." She asks me; "How would you feel about coming back next week to continue talking?" "And for the first time I think yeah maybe it is possible. Maybe…"

The psychotherapy resident has caught and shaped the affective moment between them; in this instance in time and no other. She has in Deleuze's parlance deterritorialized her engagement with medical facts and is inhabiting another plane. It is what Deleuze calls a "haecceity" which he describes as "events, incorporeal transformations that consist entirely of relations of movement and rest…capacities to affect and be affected (Deleuze & Guattari, 1987, p. 261). The trainee has opened up a new space in which to affect and be affected by moving from her psychotherapeutic framework to an indeterminate space of not knowing or explaining.

There is a shared element between the work that SPs carry out in learning and portraying roles within medical education and the work of practitioners themselves. For me, as an SP taking on a patient role, there is a productive gap. My preparation attempts to "deterritorialize" or move away from the known factual content of my story. I "court" the unknown, the uncanny. In other words it is not what I know about the case but what I do not understand or am unable to face about my story that I bring with me as the patient into a teaching encounter. For me the process is akin to creating a sculpture out of the details of patient's story....what time does she wake up? Is she in pain? How much pain? What can she no longer do that she loved to do? When I have constructed the person's physical, social, affective and historical life into a coherent whole I smash it to pieces. It is a process of wilfully forgetting the patient's story as a clinical presentation of symptoms and findings, and attending to the feelings that arise from the details of the patient's situation, her life; her relationships. I use the term "smash" to evoke the energy it takes both to create this other life as well as to throw it out. It requires abandoning certainty in order to expose oneself to unknown possibilities. In the end it is what a medical student or practicing professional and I can discover together, about the shape and texture of the pieces and how they may or may no longer fit, that takes place for me in an encounter. There is a necessary ambiguity that allows a shaping of the moment for both the SP and the interlocutor. "Acknowledging the proximity of the crack, the margins of unspeakableness, the traumatized nature of being-in-the-world and hence a great fragility is the starting point..." (Braidotti, 2006, p. 271). For the medical professional there is also a gap between the patient story and their attempt to "solve" or help the situation that they attempt to close through their words and knowledge. And sometimes through a similar "deterritorializing" – literally a moving away from a known terrain, the gap is populated as in Heather's story with the possibility of "becoming other". In this place we are far from thinking about simulation as a standardized form or mechanized representation for practice. As well the duplicity which is endemic in the relationship between SP as patient and physician is held at bay as both individuals join each other on new ground. The movement which takes place in the "between" space is affective and connected to ideas about passion and emotion.

5.3   Acting and Passion

There is an integral connection between acting and a facility with passion and affect. A doctrine of the passions, with its power to explain and illuminate the actor's art, was derived from the ancients' understanding of connections between life forces both internal and external to the human body. In early classical writings, acting was considered to endow the actor with three potencies of an enchanted kind.

> First the actor possessed the power to act on his own body. Second, he possessed the power to act on the physical space around him. Finally, he was able to act on the bodies of the spectators who shared that space with him. His expressions could transform his physical identity, inwardly and outwardly and so thoroughly that at his best he was known as Proteus (Roach, 2002, p. 26).

Such enchantments make performance a transformative and dangerous medium.

"The word passion derived from the Latin *patior* (to suffer), and suggests emotions seize upon and possess those who suffer them" (Roach 1985, p. 28). It is also the root for "compassion" – with passion. This implies that both player and audience are vulnerable to such effects. This understanding although buried in ancient lore is visible in the exalted and suspicious fascination with which those enacting roles are still viewed (famous and infamous celebrity). Power is seen to reside in an individual's ability to make others feel while at the same time being vulnerable to the effects of that power. Ahmed (2004) points out the word passion and passive share the same root in the Latin word for "suffering". She draws a link between passion/ passivity, and fear of emotionality, by which "weakness is defined in terms of a tendency to be shaped by others" (2004, p. 2). To be emotional is to have one's judgment affected. "It is to be reactive rather than active, dependent rather than autonomous and as a result, emotion needs to be harnessed by reason" (2004, p. 3).

Viewing passion as a transformative force has significance for the field of human simulation where emotion and affect are media through which knowledge is transformed into immediate lived experience. Learning that extends beyond rational and scientific explanation produces epistemological tensions. This is true for medicine, for which "malingerers", who use emotion to deceive are a scourge and detecting them as frauds a point of professional pride. Passion as an inchoate and excessive force derails objective and rational explanations. The epistemological and ontological questions raised by categorization and diagnosis of such conditions as hysteria, which I will discuss in a later section, then are tied to questions of acting as a technology of metamorphosis or mimesis with different questions about power and gender inherent in both of these possibilities.

There is a link between passion, the ascribed innate ability of women to dissemble, and attributions of women as closer to nature, ruled by appetite and less able to transcend the body through thought, will and judgment. "By identifying emotion with irrationality, subjectivity, the chaotic and other negative characteristics, and subsequently labelling women the emotional gender [...]" (Lutz, 1998, p. 54), have material implications. This is a dangerous mixture that historically has led to accusations of witch craft and views of prostitution as a natural (but unfortunate) occupation for those who have lost the battle between their natural appetites and moral social values and finds exquisite resonance in the history of women in theatre (Katritzky, 1997, p. 87).

5.4 Mapping Passion

There are links between ideas about passion as an invisible force with the potential to change oneself and others, the art of acting as a practice of shape shifting through affective techniques, and present day engagement of emotion by SPs.

The terms passion and emotion are historically mediated terms often used at different moments in attempts to understand illness as embodied, performed and socially influenced. Passion as an idea was replaced by the concept of emotion between c. 1800 and c. 1850 according to Thomas Dixon (2003). He suggests that "it was the secularization of psychology that gave rise to the creation and adoption of the new category of emotions" (p. 4).

The words 'passions' and 'affections' belonged to a network of words such as 'of the soul', 'conscience', 'fall', 'sin', 'grace', 'spirit', 'Satan', 'lower-appetite', and so on. The word 'emotions' was from the outset part of a different network of terms such as 'psychology'. 'law', observation', 'evolution', 'organism', 'brain', 'nerves', 'expression', 'behaviour', and 'viscera' (Dixon, 2003, p. 5).

Changes in ideas about passion then emerge through historical conditions, social mechanisms and political decisions, producing particular ideas about emotion as a correlate of biology. Knowledge about passion and subsequently emotion then has been sought "in the supposedly more permanent structures of human existence – in spleens, souls, genes, human nature and individual psychology [....] "(Lutz, 1998, p. 54).

A poststructuralist view of passion/emotion informs my thesis moving us beyond the biological and psychological frameworks and is aligned with Deleuze and Guattari's description of passions as "effectuations of desire" (1987, p. 399), that produce real effects in the world. They state, "Feelings become uprooted from the interiority of a subject, to be projected violently outward into a milieu of pure exteriority that lends them an incredible velocity; a catapulting force: love or hate, they are no longer feelings but affects" (Deleuze & Guattari, 1987, 356). Affect is exteriorized passion.

Passion and desire then are described by these theorists as affective forces. Affects do things, create "becomings"; the velocity of affect deterritorializes, in other words forces us into a new place. As a process that decentres the "I", passion along with emotion and affect become part of a practical ethics that encourages and works with and through difference.

5.5   Acting and Human Simulation

A number of threads need to be teased apart with respect to acting and an alternative mapping of human simulation. The first involves a discussion of different theories of acting as they formulate emotion. The earliest discussions of theatre theory in the west acknowledge a difference in beliefs about the activity of acting. As far back as the *Republic*, Plato (429-347 B.C.) described mimesis (referring to imitation) as something that occurs when the poet/rhapsode "delivers a speech as if he were someone else" (cited in Chinoy, 1970, p.6). Despite the superficial nature of the activity, it was accepted that a performer might in fact take on the qualities that he imitated …"but they should not depict or be skilful at imitating any kind of illiberality or baseness lest from imitation they should come to be what they imitate" (cited in Chinoy, 1970, p. 9). "Aristotle (384-322 B.C.) on the other hand in *Poetics,* speaks of mimesis as a performance in which the actor ceases to "speak in his own person and takes on another personality" (cited in Chinoy, 1970, p. 11). Their purpose, in essence, was to achieve a metamorphosis: a bringing someone else to presence "for by natural sympathy, they are most persuasive and affecting who are under the influence of actual passion" (Tassi, 2000, p. 5). Quintilian, (ca. 35 – ca. 100), a Roman authority on rhetoric, suggested: "Emotions should remain felt emotions but they also become impersonations [by which] I mean fictitious speeches" (Roach, 2002, p. 24).

Acknowledgement that performed emotion and affect are contagious and dangerous for both actors and audience remains a constant throughout the history of acting. Though still fascinating for theorists today, explanations now focus more on the neuroscientific rather than philosophical aspects of the phenomenon.[4]

Along the spectrum of acting techniques, styles and accompanying theories, today, performance both in theatre and outside may be viewed broadly speaking as incorporating "outside in" (mimesis) or the "inside-out" (metamorphosis) approaches. In theatre those who view acting as metamorphosis endorse what is referred to as "The Method" approach developed by Konstantin Stanislavski (1863-1938). Stanislavski formulated psychophysical techniques whereby emotions are seen as processed into art through memory, imagination and physical action (1936, p. 205). He viewed the actor's art as a rigorous process of "working on himself". As described by Stanislavski, "The creative artist feels his own life in the life of his part, and the life of his part identical with his personal life...A miraculous metamorphosis" (Stanislavski, 1936, p.269). There are a number of schools of acting whose techniques and philosophies modify and elaborate this understanding of acting, i.e., Grotowski, Strasberg. A theatre anthropologist Aldo Tassi, in his article "Performance as Metamorphosis" describes this metamorphosis as a double consciousness.

> The double consciousness which actors say takes place during the performance is a split, which takes place within the actor's consciousness. The actor finds himself identifying with someone he is not originally. What the actor does, then, when she impersonates someone is to create someone else out of herself. She brings this someone else forth from her own body. It is not a case of pretending to be someone else. It is a matter of becoming this someone else (Tassi, 2000, p. 16).

One young SP told me that she made decisions as her character about whether she would answer questions or not depending on the demeanour and tone of the students she saw (McNaughton, 2003, 2008). The character melded with the SPs experience and decision making in effect creating a new person. Along with this melding is the effect such work has on the SPs. Many SPs have spoken about lingering emotional and physical effects they experience after inhabiting roles especially intense or complex psychological ones, and the sometimes difficult time they have returning to what feels like normal (McNaughton, 1999).

Supporters of a more formal approach to acting may be seen to be taking up the views of theatre theorist Denis Diderot who developed a taxonomy of acting stages. In Le *Paradoxesur le comédien* (1830), Diderot described the successful actor as someone "who having learnt the words set down for him by the author, fools you thoroughly" (cited in Chinoy, 1970, p. 162). He believed that an actor representing an emotion must not undergo the emotion himself. "In my view…he must have in himself an unmoved and disinterested onlooker" (cited in Roach, 2002. p. 149). He explains that actors working from the heart will not be able to sustain their performance and; "Their playing is alternately strong and feeble" (cited in Roach, 2002. p. 149).

Although these theorists are not the sole authors of acting theory, SPs, both non-actors and professional actors alike, have strong opinions about whether what they are doing is a form of mimesis or metamorphosis, albeit most agree that acting as a patient opposite a person who is not an actor *per se* is very different from what occurs on stage and in film. The following discussion has relevance for enactments of illness by standardized patients today, with respect to notions about representation and performance of illness as forms of metamorphosis or mimicking and will be taken up in more detail in my examination of simulation and hysteria. Hysteria was described as a "mimicking" disorder with the allusion that its performance discredited the experience of real suffering. Acting and performance become metaphors for the "not real".

5.6 Embodied Emotion and Performance of Illness

Feminist scholars theorizing gender, and embodiment such as Alison Jaggar (1996), Elizabeth Spelman, (1989), Elizabeth Grosz (2004) Megan Boler (1999), Sarah Ahmed (2004) and others, have argued that the subordination of emotion is directly tied to the subjugation of the feminine and the body. In medicine's modernist form today, emotion is not considered "knowledge" but a non-cognitive tool placed in relationship with reason as a lesser but sometimes helpful attribute or skill. Emotion is placed, with other dualisms, such as objective/subjective, man/woman, sense/nonsense, reason/madness, rational/irrational as the lesser descriptor. It is attached to the invisible work of morality, virtue and ethics, and divided off from the "real" objective scientific work of medicine. Within discourses of illness, medical professionalism, as well as theatre, emotion is constituted as an object that can be manipulated and used as justification for particular decisions, diagnoses, and actions.

Ahmed (2004) suggests that emotions are experienced in the body as mediated by history and are part of a cultural politics. She continues:
> Focusing on emotions as mediated as well as immediate or internal, reminds us that knowledge cannot be separated from the bodily world of feeling and sensation; knowledge is bound up with what makes us sweat, shudder, tremble, all those feelings that are crucially

felt on the bodily surface, the skin surface where we touch and are touched by the world (2004, p. 171).

This idea of the porous border returns us to the "inside –out" and "outside-in" of acting and of illness as culturally mediated. For example, as will be explored in more depth a lens that views hysteria as a product of social and cultural forces represents it as a flow in both directions from physiological to psychological (inside – out) and from psychological and physiological (outside – in) with women's bodies subjected as the ultimate mediator. "In France during the late 19th century, hysteria was employed as a metaphor and became short hand for the irrational, the will-less, the uncontrollable, the convulsive, the erratic, the erotic, the ecstatic, the female, the criminal and a host of collective "Others" (Micale, 2004, p. 84).

5.7   Embodied Emotion and Performance of Social Roles

There are different theories from within the social sciences that call on theatre terminology in order to analyze the performance of social roles that occur in the day to day world through social interaction. Erving Goffman (1922-1982) wrote about social interaction, identity formation, image control and maintenance in theatrical terms of "front stage" and "back stage", "self as character". His rhetorical use of theatre terminology operated to make visible the situated and constructed aspects of public versus private personas. Arlie Hochschild, another sociologist, has studied service occupations examining gendered emotional labour inherent in different roles or parts played by workers such as stewardesses (2003). The coupling of performance as a social vehicle in tandem with the emotional aspects of performing roles whether on stage or in our everyday world has resonance for both the work in which SPs engage as teachers as well as the work of health care professionals. For the predominantly female SP field as for the still largely gendered professions of teaching and nursing, emotion work is used to reproduce normalizing expectations about practice. The ways in which various social sciences use theatre terminology metaphorically contributes to theories of professional identity as performance and are important to consider in connection with the concepts of emotion being written about within performance and theatre studies. They contribute to enriching an understanding within the health professions about how affect in involved in the social construction of identity.

5.8   An Anti- Genealogy of Human Simulation: Medicine, Charlatans, Mountebanks and Quacksalvers

In this section I am connecting the social and economic influences that have informed medicine with the emergence of SPs. The idea is that the excluded and the abject in any field are required for that field's legitimation and there is a reciprocal if not equal reliance of the official discourse on those on the fringes. Of interest for this discussion is the genealogical return, "the paradoxically surprising continuities, those echoes of counter-narratives that reverberate across time and space, waiting for the future to hear them" (Dietrich, 2007, p. xviii). Faintly audible for me are phrases that harmonize theatre and standardized patients as sites of knowledge production within medical education just as the hysterical women of Salpêtrière were for Charcot. SPs in the beginning days were mostly women and artists who were (and are today) to a large degree itinerant performers piecing together at least in part a livelihood through theatrical activity as it is applied to medical education.

Healers of all types, Shamans and Holy men and women have performed rituals of physical and spiritual healing for time immemorial, in effect engaging through affect and performance, powers of belief and persuasion as effective medicine. However, economic as well as moral considerations have informed both theatre and medicine as growing professions particularly in the West. In the fifteenth century Europe, actors and actresses supplemented their meagre incomes as itinerant performers through "quackery" or the peddling of nostrums and balms through performance.

> Increasingly recognized as central to the study of early modern medical, economic, gender and theatre history, quackery provided a way into theatre and medicine for those excluded from their official practice. Women represent the largest such category (Katritzky, 2007, p. 5).

Quacks were dismissed as pretenders to knowledge of which they are not possessed - in short, a swindler and a knave" (Katritzky. 2007, 5). While there is overlap between the work of mountebanks, charlatans and quacksalvers, all of them combine to varying degrees the three elements of medical activity, theatrical activity and itinerancy. Quacks "used theatricality, in its widest possible sense, to attract customers, promote their healing abilities, and enhance the therapeutic effects of their products" (Katritzky. 2007, p. 87). Marginalized at the edges of quack practice, women acted as accomplices (to steal from unwitting clients while having a tooth pulled) as assistants, and in some instances more overtly as prostitutes for selected male clients. Some worked as mid- wives and wise women but even here were castigated as "rusty old hags" and "female cow doctors", "deceitful tooth drawers" and "witches" (Katritzky. 2007, p. 87).

Like some of the women quacks and charlatans and mid wives who did gain access to the profession of medicine itself, a large number of women SPs have managed to use simulation as a pathway to legitimacy and power within medical education, with many in positions as Deans of medical schools and Directors of large professional programs. However for the most part, SPs do not themselves enter medicine as healers or join the ranks of University Faculty but work as itinerant performers within medicine and associated health professions.

5.8.1 SPs /Nomads

Nomadic, journey-men and women who willingly travel to take work of a diverse nature, our SPs are distant cousins to the travelling Mountebanks and Charlatans of sixteenth and seventeenth century Europe. For the large number who are not aspiring to legitimacy within medical education but rather within theatre, there is a carnivalesque overtone to the range and type of activities in which they are engaged.[5] As performers who work sporadically by virtue of their chosen field, SPs are available to help set up large venues for events, (exam sites that accommodate over 400 moving people over the course of a day), order catering, move equipment and tear down sites once they are finished as well as to act as patients over the course of these same exams. (During the SARS epidemic a recognized and successful actor was charged with pushing hospital beds up a major four lane avenue to set up a makeshift exam site.) Perpetual nomads in the Deleuzian sense of affiliation exterior to any established institutional logos, SPs it can be said "are seen to be of another species of another nature of another origin" (Deleuze and Guattari, 1987, p. 354). As performers SPs are adept at shifting affect and adapting different roles: they are irreducible to the identities which they enact, inhabiting a discomfiting location between legitimate and illegitimate worlds. This exteriority to legitimate scientific understanding is what Deleuze calls a "war machine". He states, "In every respect the war machine is of another species, another nature, another origin than the State apparatus" (Deleuze & Guattari, 1987, p. 352). (Discussion of the war machine with respect to SPs will be covered in the next chapter).

Neoliberal and modernist notions of illness, class and occupation are important for locating different kinds of patients as particular objects of medicine's gaze, and, actors as a class of patient are morally troublesome. As scavengers of human experience, actors' abilities to take on different personas and manipulate emotions can engender antipathy by those charged with their care. The spectre of malingering is never far away. And so by virtue of their location as outsiders to a profession that has need of a skill that may be used against them (malingering, or performing in excess of what is requested), SPs are in a similarly complex relationship with respect to medical education, as Charcot's hystericized women were to the discipline of neurology.

5.9   Hysteria: A Genealogical mapping

Metamorphosis, mimesis; illness, malingering; fabrication, reality; medicine and theatre and the gendered complexities of power inform a genealogy of human simulation that I argue can be traced to Charcot's theatre of incurable women in France at the end of the 19th century.

> From its origins in medicine, hysteria as word, image, theory, and diagnosis – penetrated one cultural area after another including fiction, poetry, dramaturgy, historical writing, social and political

criticism, sociology, criminology, and anthropology (Micale, 2004.p. 84).

Hysteria emerged as a crucible for Western medicine at this point in its history. "As a condition and a discursive classification it hovered between organic and psychological because it muddled the medical and the moral, [...] (were sufferers sick or shamming?)" (Porter, 1993, p. 230). Mind/body disputes highlighted by hysteria's etiology created battle lines between those who saw it as a result of pathological somatizaton and those who saw it as psychogenic (Porter, 1993, p. 235). Hysteria as an ambiguous shape shifter became a lightening rod for debates between the physiological and the imaginary. "Was hysteria just a will-o' the wisp, a fabulous or phantom? Or was it an authentic malady whose essence lay in having no essence, being prodigiously protean; the masquerading malady mimicking all others?" (Porter, 1993, p. 244). Or was it a "weapon of war" waged on an affective battleground by both patients and doctors. "The place of hysteria within the epistemology of positivist science was intensely problematic" (Micale, 2004, p. 90).

Charcot spoke of neuro-mimesis as an illness of the psyche, which resembled organic illness seen to originate in the body, with simulation as the mechanism by which one engendered pity (Porter, 1993). The idea implies that if medicine cannot locate a lesion or exact physiologically cause for signs and symptoms than the patient is malingering and enjoying power acquired through trickery. This view still holds in medicine today.[6] with hysteria now referred to by such new terms as "conversion disorder", "histrionic personality or "somataform disorder" to name a few. In instances where physiological causes are elusive illness is "psychologized" and blamed on the patient.

Theorists studying hysteria (Porter, 1993, Rousseau 1993, Showalter, 1993, Didi-Huberman, 2003, Micale, 2004) all recognize the nineteenth century as hysteria's "Belle Epoch": thanks above all to a startling emergence and convergence of mutually reinforcing conditions: a profound accentuation of the "woman question" coterminous with an evidently not unrelated expansion of organized medicine" (Porter, 1993, p. 248). Hysteria reached its zenith in an age of rapid social and cultural change and challenge to patriarchal values. "A self-renewing discourse it was capable of transforming itself both as a diagnosed disease, medical category and – linguistically – as a critique of male female relations" (Rousseau, 1993, p. xii). Modernity as an ideology of progress founded on a historical unfolding of rational principles of truth and goodness acted as a universalizing force. Its universality was based on a double pull: on the spatial level it flattened out all differences, especially the anomalous or wild ones.

Hysteria the social phenomenon was made possible and shaped by a biopolitical agenda "mapping the elements by which doctors took control of definitions of sexuality. Foucault describes the hystericization of women's bodies as one of the crucial mechanisms by which psychiatric and medical power advanced their agendas (Foucault, 1978, p.104). The emergence of the industrial state with government interest in the health of the population meant that medicine enjoyed a greater role within socio political institutions as arbiters of moral as well as physical health. Examining vast disease populations in their new public capacity, doctors made bold to become scientific policy makers for the new age. The questions they addressed – matters of hygiene, efficiency, sanity, race, sexuality, morality, criminality, liability and so forth – were inevitably morally charged. "Psychiatry blossomed colonizing its own location in asylums, and the University polyclinics" (Porter, 1993, p. 248).

Particular techniques of authority were produced in order to shape and ultimately control invisible urges and desires. Emotional and or sexual "internal disposition" were made visible through specialized practices such as technologies of surveillance and confession. Both sexuality and emotion at this time are constructed as part of an individual's physiologically makeup. As objects, emotion and sex are considered measurable along a continuum from normal to abnormal providing subject positions for those measuring and those needing to be measured. Scientific claims based on psychometric judgments become accepted truths providing evidence for classification of individuals and population management systems. Institutional power takes shape as the locus of regulation and reform because sex and emotion are not only physiological traits but are also mutable through educative and therapeutic processes.

5.10 Hysteria and Simulation

> You will meet with simulation at every step....and one finds himself sometimes admiring the amazing craft, sagacity, perseverance which women under the influence of the great neurosis will put in play for purposes of deception – especially when the physician is made to be the victim (Gilman, 1993, p. 352).

My interest here is not in reiterating hysteria, a well researched area taken up importantly by feminist theorists committed to demystifying gender and social control encoded in women's diseases, "(especially the hysteria diagnosis in the age of Freud)" (Rousseau, 1993, p. viii). My intent is rather to inquire into acting as a counter narrative which has "come to be appropriated by and made appropriate for dominant institutional knowledges" (Diedrich, 2007, p. xx). How have ideas about emotion, gender and theatre in 19th century France made possible the work in which SPs engage today?

There are striking parallels to be drawn between the performance of hysteria in J.M. Charcot's Salpêtrière "living museum of pathology" of the nineteenth century and the work of actors portraying patient stories in the twenty first. To start, both Charcot credited with "inventing" and establishing hysteria and its sufferers as "Stars of hysteria", and Barrows credited as the father of simulated patients, were neurologists. Although I am not interrogating claims about their work it is interesting that as neurologists they are the "fathers" of systems of standardization and performance employing living "actresses" for the purposes of teaching about particular physiological signs. As mentioned in the introduction, my narrative represents a separate trajectory for human simulation, an anti-genealogy that calls in part on the emergence of the anatamo-clinical method, the operation of bio-power and on theories of subjectification outlined in the writing of Foucault.

5.10.1. Simulating Hysteria

Hysteria was referred to by Charcot as "la grandesimulatrice". It was considered the" mimic disorder" with "the problem of simulation as a kind of art for its own sake (l'art pour l'art), done with the idea of making a sensation to excite pity" (Porter, 1993, p. 280). Described as a kind of burlesque, hysteria may also be read as a duplicitous seduction: were not the patients or their diseases duping the scientific, voyeuristic doctors? (Showalter, 1993, p. 257). The predominantly working class women (four thousand of them) confined within he walls of Salpêtrière in the last few decades of the nineteenth century were regarded with hostility and denounced as "veritable actresses" (Showalter, 1993,302); a sinister assignation denoting intentional manipulation. Hysterical women were interpreted as naturally duplicitous, liars and manipulators, quick learners adept at emotional mimicry and performance and in control of emotion as an instrument to get what they want, while also being seen as victims to uncontrollable urges who needed to be tamed, and managed for the good of society.

Didi- Huberman suggested that a "reciprocity of charm was instituted between physicians with their insatiable desire for images of hysteria, and, hysterics who willingly participated and actually raised the stakes through their increasingly theatricalized bodies" (Didi-Huberman, 2003, p. xi).The "charm" is gendered and interrogates the idea of emotional excess and sexuality as a feminine control issue. The gendered history of hysteria as a women's disorder is a double edged sword that allows no escape and returns the rationale of the witch hunts. Foucault suggests through his description of the "hystericization of women's bodies", that women at this time in history were interpreted as "thoroughly saturated with sexuality" (Foucault, 1978/1980, p. 104). "The hysterical seizure was regarded as an acting out of the female experience, as spasm of hyper-femininity, mimicking both childbirth and the female orgasm" (Showalter, 1993, p. 287). Whether interpreted as prone to over excitation or repression, women were seen as victims of their sexuality, inciting the necessity for focused attention by newly formed medical specialties (gynecology became a specialty during this time) and complexes of power inaugurated through a privileging of visual representation.

5.10.2 Hysteria as Theatre

There were fruitful connections between the arts and medicine during the "Belle Epoch" in France during which time the links "between the arts and psychiatry were closer than those between the arts and any other branch of medicine" (Micale, 2004, p.17). Charcot inspired paintings, novels, and plays as well as extensive commentary in the press. This interplay between scientific and cultural discourses Micale argues did not move simply uni-directionally from science to the arts but that the arts largely influenced and were part of the constitution of scientific perspectives related to illness.

An unprecedented intersection of theatre and medicine took place at this time finding both inspiration and expression within the hospital clinics of Salpêtrière and Charcot's Tuesday Lectures. A new genre, *le théâtre medical* was created by André de Lorde with plays entitled: "Obsession", "The Laboratory of Hallucinations", and "Crime in an Insane Asylum" (Gordon, 2004, p. 95). Alfred Binet, an eminent experimental psychologist wrote five and possibly eight plays for the Grande Guignol and Joseph Babinsky collaborated on plays with such titles as "The Mad One" and "Theatre of Fear" (Gordon, 2004, p. 95).

In this milieu the hysterical heroine flourished. "In 1884 when Sarah Bernhardt wanted to perfect her performance of the attack of hysterical insanity in the play *Adrienne Lecouvreur,* she repaired for practice to a cell in the quartiers des aliénés at Salpêtrière" (Micale. 2004, p. 76). And "more than one of Charcot's patients "cured" or not, went on to make a living as a street singer, or, in the case of Jane Avril as a Moulin Rouge dancer, when he or she left the hospital" (Gordon, 2004, p. 94). Charcot's

Tuesday Lectures were theatre spectaculars. Described by one visiting Swedish doctor Axel Muenthe,

> ...when the huge amphitheatre was filled to the last place with a multicoloured audience drawn from tout Paris, authors, journalists, leading actors and actresses, fashionable demimondaines the hypnotized women patients put on a spectacular show before this crowd of curiosity seekers (Showalter, 1993, p. 311).

Didi-Huberman goes so far as to suggest that "The Tuesday Lectures moreover, are written, or rather rewritten, just like plays with lines, soliloquies, stage directions, asides by the hero and so on" (Didi-Huberman, 2003, p. 243). This reference is footnoted and ascribed to Charcot's notebook *Leçons du mardi (1887-1888) and Leçons du mardi (1888 – 1889)*. I believe Didi-Huberman was writing metaphorically referring to the power relations in which the doctor demonstrating phases of hysterico epilepsy with a hypnotized subject is like a director who is in full possession of the passage from one scene to the next. Didi-Huberman returned to the "voracious dramaturgical passion of the physicians of Salpêtrière and their *desire to have all the roles played...*" (emphasis in the original), as responsible for generating interest in the effect of hypnotic experimentation on the hysterical subject, or as he refers to the patients as *subject[s] of simulation"* (Didi-Huberman, 2003, p. 228). There is convergence between the use of hypnotized hysterics and standardized patients as instruments of research and inquiry beyond their pedagogical usefulness. The intersections of power that operate in these instances rest on questions of representation - as a doubling of that which exists (in the case of the hysterical patients) or performance - as a fabrication of that which does not (in the case of SPs) Is it metamorphosis or mimesis? Is it really felt or simply mimed?

> The hysterics of Salpêtrière were so "successful" ...as *subjects of mimesis* that, in the eyes of the physicians who had become directors of their fantasies, they entirely lost their status as *subjects of distress* (Didi-Huberman, 2003, p. 229).

Where does this leave the patient who is both the centre of attention as star attraction and mimicking imposter?

5.10.3 Complicity/Performance

I suggest that the relationship between theatre and medicine is one of complicity as was the case in the nineteenth century, "For hysteria is the classic disease of the imagination not of the uterus – as Charcot and Freud understood" (Gilman, 1993, p. 359). The explicit power relations and highly sexualized readings of hysteria within Charcot's hospital produced complex unions in which all parties were held hostage by virtue of the stakes each performance represented. For Charcot the correct performance by the patient was crucial to his reputation, for in demonstrating the repeatability of the course of a hysterico-epileptic seizure through physical induction he was establishing it as a positive scientific disorder with specific location, causes, signs and possible treatments. "This particular theatre is also the theatre of classification of words, the classification of subjects: it is the theatre of power, of fabricating taxonomies of suffering bodies" (Didi-Huberman, 2003, p.244). And "when the event is spontaneous it must be checked, it must be methodically reprovoked. It is a theatricality that searches for a kind of crystallization of the aspect in theory – a refabrication of evidence" (Didi-Huberman, 2003, p. 244). A similar crystallization through standardization was the main impetus behind the creation of "standardized" patients as a technology. This will be explored in the next section.

For the seemingly powerless patient, there were stakes indicating that they had control of something they might not have completely appreciated but knew was important. In Augustine's case study description, allusion is made to her having the benefit of different clothes to wear for the different scenes she enacted as well as freedom to walk the grounds (Showalter, 1993, p. 312), perhaps freedom and special treatment for appropriate performances. Patients such as Blanch Wittman and Augustine were referred to as the "Stars of Hysteria" for a good reason. They were able to reliably perform the required sequence of events in such as a way as to validate Charcot's ideas and procedures. "The hysteria that Charcot studied – or, better perhaps, that he and his patients co-produced – was a palimpsest of a performance, many layered with meanings" (Porter, 1993, p. 256).

According to Diderot, reflection is the second stage in the three-stage process of developing an internal (psychological) model that the actor uses in assuming a role. During reflection "the observed facts of emotional behaviour…which have been stored in the actor's memory are recombined in the imagination as a sequence of passions appropriate to the character type he enacts" (Roach, 1985, p.141). He continues, "Reflection together with observation and practice he explains is why the great actor can perform consistently from day to day: the blueprint remains before the mind's eye to be called on from an emotional distance" (p. 141). Were the patients acting "from an emotional distance?" Or were they transforming themselves from within a complex of physiologically experienced sensations? These questions echo those still being asked by SPs engaged in performing patients' stories today.

5.10.4 Representation/Performance/Simulation/Acting: The Invisible Made Visible

The following discussion will explore the role of representation and performance in the constitution of hysteria as a discursive object and subject position and as a precursor to the field of human simulation. I suggest that discourses constituting "representation" as a stand in for "real, and "performance" as a stand in for the "not real", blur the boundaries between disease as the property of physicians or patients' embodied illness experiences. Such confusion is generative, producing new forms of knowledge, positions of authority, objects and spaces both literal and ontological.

Photography was a powerful new tool in the 19th century. "Indeed photography was born at a moment when not only the end of history but the advent of absolute knowledge were awaited" (Didi-Huberman, 2003, p. 30). For the medical scientist it was simultaneously an experimental procedure (laboratory tool), a museological procedure (scientific archive) and a teaching procedure (a tool of transmission) (2003, p.30). It had indexical value as evidence. The generation of photographs, charts and performances constituted as real that which was visible, privileging the medical gaze and authorizing physicians as authorities on decoding physical signs and behaviours as stigmata of inner turmoil. The art of photography as well as the science constituted hysteria as an object of knowledge and provided the means by which its particular features became known. "The medium of representation – photography, live demonstrations, shaped the image of the illness" (Didi-Huberman, 2003, p. 120). As a site of scientific representation, hysteria had no coherent or fixed identity of its own. The camera was important; a crucial tool for the invention of hysteria capturing physical behaviours as inimitable proof its physiological basis.

"Hysteria was not a simple copy or representation of another "real" pathological type. Its appropriate metaphor was less a mirror than a hall of mirrors or echo chamber" (Micale, 2004, p. 90). Such ambiguity motivated scientists to attempt to distil its essence into a constant. Like SPs today, the stars of Charcot's "hysteria theatre", were valued for their ability to represent at will, (not their own), visually in a repeatable manner the specific features and phases of a particular illness. Elaborate mechanisms were put in play to standardize, capture, visually document, classify and freeze hysteria's signs as cardinal and universal. The repeatability and regularity of patient's attitudes was important to justify the positivist claims to a physiological location and cause for hysteria. "There was a veritable industry of standardization and measurement of every act of perception imaginable and unimaginable" (Didi-Huberman, 2003, p. 130). Together through photography, theatre and spectacle, hysteria was constituted as a physiologically explainable disorder; a ghostly projection, a product of duplicity and complicity.

5.10.5　Duplicity/Representation – Complicity/Performance

I am sitting in a wheel chair in my blue hospital gown waiting in a hallway outside the main amphitheatre. I had undergone laparoscopic back surgery the previous week and I could have been convalescing at home, however was waiting "in the wings" to be presented by my neurosurgeon during morbidity and mortality (M & M) rounds. On discovering that I worked as a standardized patient early on in our relationship my neurosurgeon became fascinated with the idea of presenting me as an anomalous case of neurological damage to his colleagues. I was requested to enact a spontaneous "Marching Jacksonian" seizure. In order to learn how to do this I remained in the hospital as a patient for a week, visited by my doctor daily with various heavy text books full of pictures and large unfamiliar words. This was seen as a privilege. I surely wouldn't have received any such attention had I not agreed to this performance. The coaching consisted of his answering questions about what the various symptoms look like when they occur, timing, rate, duration…How does it start? Where does it start? How fast a progression up the body? Is it symmetrical? How long does the attack take to subside? What is the specific nature of the tremors? This was a long time ago and I know I wondered about the ethics of what I was doing but also remember feeling perplexed. I was on my back in a bed in a gown and this surgeon had just successfully taken me out of over two years of debilitating pain. Did I owe this to him? Was I being included in a matrix of power that made me special? Was I being recognized for my skills as an SP? The complex of power relations so evident to me now were lost on me at this point in my life.

I am wheeled in to the auditorium full of physicians. My CT scans and "real" patient files had been presented and I, as the anomaly, was to answer questions regarding my symptoms (onset duration, intensity, and associated symptoms). Within a few minutes of the questioning I began the seizure starting at my right foot (my surgery had been on the left side) and progressing with fine tremors up my body including my neck and head and finishing with my right hand. I had no idea if in fact this was right or not. The effect on the audience was palpable. There was immediately a buzz and some concern for my well being and then an onslaught of questions (which I didn't really know how to answer.) Then the esteemed neurosurgeon said something like April Fools! and things became very heated. As you can imagine there were those who were fascinated at the theatrical possibility that they had just witnessed while others were horrified at having been "outed" (for believing the performance) and betrayed by one of their own colleagues.

I recently spoke to a man whose mother - a family doctor - had been in the audience that day and he recalled his mother's upset. She found the ethical issues raised by the presentation more troublesome than any other aspect. Duplicity, trust, power, theatre are intertwined. I was both a patient and an actor on that day and through my duplicity and complicity tapped into medicine's deep professional fear of incompetence – of not being able to discern the "real" from the "fake". I made them *feel* for me in a way that was based on misinformation. I crossed a sacrosanct professional boundary, one that defends against duplicity in order to be able to trust observations but more importantly feelings as the ethical basis for patient/doctor relationships.

5.11 Conclusion

In this chapter I have examined the relationships between acting, illness, and emotion and linkages with the arts and hysteria as a possible counter memory in the genealogy of standardized patients. By including aesthetic and cultural considerations in the examination such a mapping provides a more inclusive and multi dimensional reading of the field of human simulation.

As mentioned in the introduction, SPs gain legitimacy both as actors and educators through their expertise in the performance of clinical representation. There are attendant pressures to perform as the "good patient" meaning doubly the compliant performer, according to both a clinical idea of the illness and a physicians' interpretation of the patient's experience. This takes on many forms of both *dissimulation*, or hiding that which is present, such as ideas, feelings and expressions about their experience while in role, as well as *simulation* – enacting that which is not present, which often involves kinds of responses (a certain kind of anger or sadness) counter to what in actuality would be the person's reaction. For SPs then, as for the hysterics of Salpêtrière, duplicity and complicity in performing "good patients" produces and reproduces a particular construction of the "good doctor".

Paradoxically perhaps when talking about acting with SPs who are professional actors, they insist that what they are doing when portraying a patient is "not acting" "It is insulting", one individual told me, "to have the student or teacher tell me after an interview that I was such a good actor, because I cried or something." There is the implication in this comment that acting means "not real" and furthermore fake and therefore not "good acting" even to the actors themselves. It is not about the character but about what happens in the flash of exchange between individual bodies. I think that the word "acting" complicates our understanding of the intentions and power dynamics that are different between acting a role (from a disinterested location?) and acting a certain way to gain something personally whether attention, drugs or, respect for your skill as an educator using acting as a medium (interested location). An SP's location in fact straddles the interested location of a teacher who wants to be respected for their investment in the educational activity (they are not pretending for their own sake) and the disinterested location of the actor (doing a good job at making you feel something). This investment is tied not so much to the actual story itself (I think unlike a real patient) but to the effect they are having on their student/audience in their enactment and the learning which may emerge as a result.

Were the hysterical women "acting" in a way that is parallel to SPs? In a similar manner the boundaries are blurred. The need to represent a story as signs and symptoms, whether it is your own story or you are living inside it for a time, privileges the one who is gazing. In the case of the women hysterics in Salpêtrière who perhaps enacted both patient and fake patient in order to gain the help they needed, as "perpetually possible" patient were they duplicitous, or complicitous? It is not about "real" or "not real" but about how well your story is performed according to a particular set of rules and expectations. When the effect of the interaction is the focus it is a cat and mouse game in which the narcissism of the practitioner not the actor is protected by a "correct" portrayal. If the patient or ironically, the SP is identified as "acting", even "well done", it has material implications. It is experienced as a failure that cuts across professional and personal boundaries. As one SP said to me "How do they know that it isn't true…that I haven't really had this experience and know what it feels like?"

Charcot had a professional stake in how hysteria was defined and accepted within 19th century medicine which was played out over debates of physiology and psychology. The complex of power that inflects the relations between doctor and teaching patients is visible in what Didi-Huberman (2003) describes as "…an extraordinary complicity between patients and doctors, a relationship of desires, gazes, and knowledge" (p. xi) based on what the hysterics of Salpêtrière could exhibit with their bodies.

A genealogy of hysteria as a form of theatre constituted by medicine's "insecure but ambitious agenda" (Porter, 1993, p. 236) during the mid nineteenth century creates a counter-memory that helps us think differently about the historical and practical conditions shaping standardized patients and the work in which they engage as educators and actors. The instrumental use of human performance as a form of evidence returns me to my own work of human simulation within medical education. This is not a heroic or linear undertaking but a critical and ethical intervention which attempts to "recognize the political implications underpinning the categories, concepts, theories, epistemologies and methods of positing objects and relations" (Foucault, 1972, p. 202).

Notes

1. My great appreciation to L.J. Nelles for our many conversations about the connections between hysteria and the work of SPs.

2. The painting is Jacques-Joseph Moreau de Tours. *Hysterics of the Charité on the Service of Dr. Luys* (1890) Bethseda Md.: National Library of medicine. In Gilman S. "Hysteria, Feminism and Gender" in S. Gilman *Hysteria Beyond Freud*. University of California Press. Berkeley, Los Angeles, London. p. 348.

3. "Charcot's clinic was noted for the large number of female patients who, under hypnosis, produced spectacular attacks of *grandehystérie* or "hystero-epilepsy" a prolonged and elaborate convulsive seizure. The attack could be induced or relieved by pressure on certain areas of the body- what Charcot called *hysterogenic* zones – and these were especially to be found in the ovarian region. A complete seizure involved three phases: the epileptoid phase in which the patient lost consciousness and foamed at the mouth; the phase of "clownism" (Charcot was a great fan of the circus), involving eccentric physical contortions; and the phase of *"attitudes passionnelles,"* or sexual poses. The attack ended with a back-bend called the *arc-en-cercle*" Showalter E. (1993) "Hysteria, Feminism and Gender" in S. Gilman *Hysteria Beyond Freud*. University of California Press. Berkeley, Los Angeles, London. p. 307-308.

4. See McConachie, B. (2007). Falsifiable Theories for Theatre and Performance Studies. *Theatre Journal*. 59. 553-577: in which he cites a theory of "visual intentionalism". Developed by Pierre Jacob and Marc Jeannerod, the theory posits that an audience response to

actor affect is related to the interaction of two visual systems that are below consciousness and which are physiologically predetermined.... a dual model of human visual processing that works differently when one is thinking about the inanimate world than when one is watching others act in intentional ways. (561) Four major claims are made by P. Niedenthal et al (2005) in a further study. Important for the practice of medicine and the use of simulation in teaching medical students are: 1) "embodied emotions produce corresponding subjective emotional states in the individual,", and 2) while imagining other people and events also produces embodied emotions and corresponding feelings. (McConachie, 2007, 562)"

5. The University of Toronto SP program may represent an anomalous experience with respect to its operations. It functions as a large self supporting not for profit educational enterprise within the Faculty of Medicine. It exists in the "white spaces" of the University governance structures with changeable reporting relationships. This has meant that a fiercely guarded independence and autonomy has grown as a cultural survival strategy. The artists, educators and administrators experience a community that is akin to bonds that form in itinerant theatre companies and on film sets in which creativity, possibility and inventiveness are valued. While those working in the more "technical" medical simulation world are sometimes referred to as "boys with toys", the women educators in the standardized patient field have been referred to as "the SP ladies" or more derogatorily as "the washing women of medical education"

for their often multiple roles of organizing and cleaning up after educational events.

6. See *My Imaginary Illness: A Journey into Uncertainty and Predjudice in Medical Diagnosis.* By Chloe G. K. Atkins, 2010. ILR Press, Ithica and London. p. 348

Chapter 6 Standardized Patients, the State, and the Nomad War Machine

6.0   Introduction

In this chapter I read the work of SPs and their relations within medical education through the lens of Deleuze and Guattari's a *thousand plateaus*, specifically their *Treatise on Nomadology:-The War Machine*. The centrality of affect as an unacknowledged material force and the systems of signification and representation that locate SPs in an exteriorized relationship to medicine suggest Deleuze and Guattari's thesis regarding the war machine and the State. Deleuze and Guattari offer me a lens and an alternative ontology which they call *nomodology* (1987, p. 43), through which to read differently the work of SPs. My reading is an anti-genealogy that maps ruptures and discontinuities but also linkages and "assemblages of desire", connections that become visible as intensities and speeds and which challenge taken for granted notions about the stability of identity, knowledge, reality and difference. Movement is inherent in the physical, institutional and affective dimensions of the field of human simulation. Deleuze and Guattari's theory of "nomad/war machines" offers a conceptual language and framework through which to unpack and repack the various forces and relations shaping SP work.

As in the previous chapter I am "mapping" my understanding of SPs, following connections rhizomatically – that is - in a non linear and ultimately generative movement. "The map has to do with performance, whereas the tracing always involves alleged competence" (Deleuze & Guattari, 1987, p. 12-13). In other words I am not reproducing knowledge and analysis through tracing over in order to arrive at a stable referent or answer but rather following lines that connect in "strange new ways" in order to create the story of standardized patients as unimagined producers of knowledge and experience. In engaging Deleuze and Guattari's rhizomatic analysis I outline possibilities that include a potential for an explicit and embodied ethics of practice based on compassion. As an embodied practice such an ethics entails "a play of complexity binding the cognitive to the emotional, the intellectual to the affective and connecting them all to a socially embedded ethics of sustainability" (Braidotti, 2006, p. 156). My intention is to contribute to new understanding about the SP professionalizing project while effecting creative possibilities fundamentally unaddressed in any literature on SPs from inside or outside the field.

6.1 The State and royal science

> It is in terms not of independence but of co-existence and competition in a perpetual field of interaction, that we must conceive of interiority and exteriority, war machines of metamorphosis and State apparatuses of identity, bands, kingdoms, megamachines and empires (Deleuze & Guattari, 1987 p. 360-361).

The line that follows standardized patients as a possible technology within medical simulation technologies – a path from the aeronautic "blue box link trainer", through military and nuclear industrial concerns to medical education – brings us to a particular conception of standardized patients which is embedded in the name itself and manifest in many of the activities in which they are engaged. This is not better or worse than other ways in which SPs are understood and used, but locates them in particular relational matrix to medical education and the profession of medicine itself.

Medicine in Deleuze and Guattari's treatise can be seen as a "royal science" tied to the concerns of "State" which delineates an entire system of thought, science, philosophy and action. As described by Deleuze and Guattari royal science is delineated by templates, rules and legislated reason in the support of State sanctioned goals. I suggest that SPs are essentially exterior to this world and their involvement in it presents both risks and rewards. In this telling SPs are Deleuze and Guattari's original "nomad/ war machine" with respect to the "Royal science" of medicine and through their activities and alliances within medical education, deterritorialize and reterritorialize knowledges within assemblages of emotion and affect.

> A distinction must be made between two types of science or scientific procedures: [Royal science] consists in "reproducing," the other [nomad science] in "following." Royal science organizes itself according to templates, reason and goals. Whereas a nomad science seems to "develop eccentrically following flows and singularities of matter (Deleuze & Guattari, 1987, p. 372).

Although Deleuze and Guattari posit an antagonism and competition between the interiority of the State and its royal science and the exteriorized nomad war machine, I am not setting up an ideological dichotomy here between the state and the worker nor am I employing a Foucauldian critique of power/knowledge/truth, but rather negotiating theoretically in the "between" space. At the limit all that counts is the constantly shifting borderline (Deleuze & Guattari, 1987, p.367). Deleuze and Guattari separate themselves from Foucault in their conception of desire and affect as productive and creative of reality. Unlike Foucault, Deleuze and Guattari conceptualize power as secondary to desire which they see as "purely affirmative and not a desire to resist another force" (Best &Kellner, 1991, p.101). I am then following Deleuze and Guattari in examining the relationship between two forces – the State and the war machine -- through an alternate ontology, which they call a nomodology that recognizes movement of all kinds (physical, affective, institutional) as constitutive of knowledges and different realities.

6.1.1 OSCE training

Twelve of us sit around a table, "recruited" to portray a patient case for one station in an Objective Structured Clinical Examination. It is for a high stakes licensing examination in which hundreds of "candidates" from across Canada will perform as "doctors to be" in a series of five and ten minute SP stations over the course of a day. Immediately evident is the similarity between all of us in the room. We are all white women of the same approximate age, height and weight in a training session for a five minute physical examination station. As lay people we are engaging with a specific assemblage here in which acting meets military order and discipline.

We are all given the patient case to read over. It consists of a number of bullet points on a page which are organized according to the clinical examination template: Inspection, auscultation, palpation, percussion etc. with our history organized likewise into Chief complaint, history of present illness, duration, location, intensity, quality of pain, aggravating and alleviating symptoms etc…We train to the checklist[1], in other words, we all become this patient and respond to query and touch only in so much as it fits into the medical template that is used to assess the candidate and nothing more. Our history is delivered in sound bites that are as similar to each other as possible. This is the first priority of training for OSCEs; ensuring that the quantity and quality of exchange whether verbal, physical (expressions of pain) or affective is standardized. It is a "cat and mouse" game which we play out with our Trainer. "Can you tell me more about the pain you are experiencing?" We respond: "What do you mean?" Trainer: "I mean you have told me that you have x pain. Can you tell me a bit more about it?" SP: "Um, it really hurts." This agreed upon non informational exchange is considered necessary in order to force "candidates" to be specific about their questioning so that they can "get" the checklist mark, i.e., "Asks about the quality of the pain." (SP response: "Sharp") *Check*. If I as an SP just told my story without these rules in place, the observing examiner[2] would not be able to reward the candidate with the appropriate check marks. Standardizing the responses in this way it is suggested, is in the best interests of the candidates, offering them all the same opportunities to get marks. It is not easy work for SPs to reward closed ended questions and respond to various qualities of touch ("Was that deep or shallow palpation?") repeated every five minutes for a possible thirty two – sixty-four times over the course of a day.

We are building an assemblage of becoming–doctor and fixed–patient that is premised on both established content knowledge and physical exam skills: the "what" (knowledge) and the "how" (skill). Affect that is acceptable or "appropriate", and by this I am referring not only to the expression of emotion but to the energy and intensity that is released "between" bodies, is hooked to a predetermined checklist item. It is grounded and contained.

Deleuze and Guattari make a distinction between the tool and the weapon with respect to their function and effect. In this examination assemblage the SP is the tool, not the weapon which will be examined later in the chapter, and is in relation to the candidate and the examiner as a captured force that is put to use. "Linear displacement from one point to another constitutes the absolute movement of a tool, but it is the vortical absolute occupation of space that constitutes the absolute movement of the weapon" (Deleuze & Guattari, 1987, p. 397). As can be seen from an OSCE training protocol SPs as tools are a consequence of a particular royal science assemblage in the profession of medicine.

6.1.2 OSCE and the State

The first tenet or "O" for Objective" in OSCE is related to fairness as it relates to providing the same opportunity for all candidates so they have the same experience as a result of establishing standardized and controllable circumstances. Observed performance assessments rest on a neo-liberal conception of the individual as the lone agent and sole creator of success. Ideas such as "fairness" and "objectivity" when tied to OSCEs make invisible the very structures that isolate the candidate and future "doctor to be" within a matrix of power relations, in a reproductive rather than generative possible future. They isolate and defend (decisions, actions) rather than connect and generate. The OSCE station assemblage of "Candidate –SP–Examining Doctor" is a machine that belongs to the State and its need to have a "limitative distribution and hierarchical ranking (the measurement of the degree of perfection of a term's self resemblance in relation to a supreme standard, man, god, or gold: value, morality)" (Massumi, 1987, p. xi-xii). The idea of objectivity permeates all aspects of OSCE activity, producing objects such as: SP training protocols to ensure standardized performances, checklists to make sure that there is a reliable grid on which to measure individual candidate performance, as well as, timing systems to control for interaction with the "case". This system allows for comparison between and across, candidate, station, school, geography, race, gender, etc through psychometrics – an applied statistical grid. It erases difference of all kinds such as age, race, (dis)ability ethnicity in the requirement that the tool be standardized.

For Deleuze and Guattari "State" is another word for representational thinking which "reposes on a double identity: of the thinking subject and of the concepts it creates and to which it lends its own presumed attributes of sameness and constancy. Its concern is to establish a correspondence between these symmetrically structured domains" (Massumi, 1987, p. xi). Vocabulary related to OSCEs such as candidates, recruitment, training protocols, standardization, tracks, circuits, stations, security, are analogic to a military order that supports the State in meeting its needs through establishing set lines, paths and its striating of mental space. In OSCEs, fairness in the form of illusionary objectivity is accompanied by equally elusive security practices and measures. Signed confidentiality forms, protocols for leaked checklists, and measures to catch cheaters are all part of a containment that produces a specific kind of movement that is both limited and limiting – it is limiting in its parts which are assigned constant directions are oriented in relation to one another, divisible by boundaries and can interlink and reproduces itself as justice, truth and rational order" (Deleuze & Guattari, 1987, p.382).

The "S" for the "structured" part of OSCE is an entrenched space, striated and gridded along a flat surface confined as by gravity to a horizontal plane. Physically, enactments in multiple five and ten minute encounters, temporally signalled by buzzers, arrayed across "tracks" and circuits" necessitate confinement to "fixed paths in well defined directions, which restrict speed, regulate circulation, relativise movement and measure in detail the relative movements of subjects and objects" (Deleuze & Guattari, 1987, p. 386). But also affectively our standardized representations are confined to a closed space limited to "predictable "accurate and reproducible arrangements. According to Deleuze and Guattari's nomadology such a space is attached to the "logos"; of entrenching oneself in closed space (hold the fort), but which I think in this instance is perhaps also "hold the gate" with respect to those being allowed into the royal profession of medicine. The OSCE machine serves the State through "reducing the many to the One of identity and ordering them by rank" (Massumi, 1987, p. xiii). This describes the function of checklists which act in conjunction with SPs, as tools of discrimination between candidates in the interests of the profession. "The ideal of reproduction, deduction, or induction as part of royal science ... treats differences of time and place as so many variables, the constant form of which is extracted precisely by the law" (Deleuze & Guattari, 1987, p.372). The OSCE is the reproductive machine for the royal science of Medicine.

Medical education is a clinical world ("C" of OSCE) in which SPs have always been outsiders, signalled very effectively by anachronistic practices, such as not telling the SP what condition they were training for or portraying. Sometimes not even the trainer was allowed to know the clinical picture being presented. The clinical meaning and logic of a patient presentation weren't considered relevant information for an SP who only needed to provide the necessary responses in an interaction. In other words why I was having a pain was not something I as the SP needed to know. The other rationale for such omissions was that SPs, being lay people, presented a risk. They could not be trusted to withhold the "answer" or diagnosis from the candidate and possibly reduce the differential power of the exam checklist. For example, in the exam training described above the SPs were learning from a paper case that omitted details of the patient's story that might distract from the information deemed important for the encounter. "Pertinent negatives", were and, still are included in order that SPs don't misdirect through misinformation. However the rule is, if you don't know the answer to the question the answer is "no" or "I don't know". There is right information to gather in OSCEs and even though the SPs don't necessarily know what it is they need to be vigilant about not leading the examinee astray.

As mentioned earlier, a bullet form or very shallow story often provided no information regarding diagnosis, prognosis or effective management, only what was to be performed. Ironically it was felt that this would keep the portrayal more "real" as patients don't usually visit their doctors with full understanding of what is going on. I say ironically because this lack of information led, in my experience, to whacky and wonderful interpretations and digressions from SPs portraying the same case, who like "real" patients put information and experiences together in distinct ways. So rather than having the effect of controlling for and standardizing responses, the absence of information actually proliferated creativity. This resulted in making SPs seem more "real" perhaps but pointing up the fact that the "real" that SPs are supposed to be in fact does not equate with patient experiences. In fact it does not even equate with physicians' ideas about their patients (who surely create explanations for themselves in the absence of information?), but rather represent a monstrous hybrid that belongs to OSCEs and medical education alone.

The result is a "becoming – not patient" who is not a real patient but rather is tied to a closed system of possible responses residing in a reductive reproduction of similarity. Epistemic violence takes place in the homogenization of representations in which unknown "others" are rendered as the self's shadow" (Diedrich, 2007, p. 103). Affectively neutered, the shadows that SPs enact as "becoming not-patient" belong to the "double dead" not unlike a cadaver used for dissection in which there is no interior that matters beyond its generalizability and universalizing function (Belling, 2009 as cited in Nelles 2011).

There has been a shift over the years from this paternalistic practice mostly for the reasons mentioned above; that limiting information to those portraying patients did not in effect lead to greater accuracy. Also through years of experience SPs are now experts in exam logistics, administration, SP training, exam blueprinting, case, and checklist development and are taking part in exam case development which has democratized the process somewhat. The most prevalent assemblage still involves clinicians together with psychometricians creating OSCEs based on a rational foundation of order, especially for high stakes assessments. However, assemblages of other sorts are created through different alignments of force. This change signals a "territorialization" of SPs to royal science as experts in transforming medical events and clinical details into enactments in which SPs inhabit the "between" of "not-knowing patient" and "knowing-too much SP".

6.2 Emotion Affect and Assessment Assemblages

In the assemblage of SP and OSCE, emotion is constructed as interior to the subject, to be excavated as feeling that is representative of a form. "The angry patient", "the borderline personality disorder," "the grieving widow" all have specific intensities of response as well as content that serve as items on a checklist. For example the borderline personality disordered patient may need to challenge the sincerity of a candidate's desire to help with a statement like, "Look me in the eye and tell me that you really care!" Both pathologized and turned into diagnostic fodder, affect and emotion are tied to expectations about candidates' appropriate responses that can be plotted on a checklist. For example, in an exam station in which the patient is insulting or angry, there may be a checklist item regarding the candidate's ability to manage their own emotions in response to being insulted or yelled at. There is always a goal or right answer and as such there is an attempt to subordinate the positive turbulence of affect to a linear movement between two points; a line that can be analyzed, and named with the intent of reproducing it. For instance, portraying a patient with schizophrenia in nine minutes according to a checklist created to assess a candidate's ability to: collect information, ascertain level of functioning and "manage" the patient's affect, illustrates the reductive effect such a configuration has on anything but the most rudimentary of possible affective exchanges. Such proscribed exchanges construct professional expectations about possible affective and emotional connections as instrumental and limited.

In this analysis OSCEs, both in their form and their role within medical education are what Deleuze and Guattari refer to as royal science. Royal science which is essential to State thought then aspires to universality, and "involves reproduction, iteration, and reiteration… in which iteration is reduced to a modality of technology or of the verification of science" (Deleuze & Guattari, 1987, p. 372). It arrays itself on a plane of formation and organization in an endlessly reproductive relationship to its own dissemination and identity. OSCEs form one assemblage within which SPs are brought into relationship to Royal science as a reproductive technology. However, there are others that work at different levels of organization proliferating possibilities in strange and unexpected ways much like our own Standardized Patient Program.

This is not a totalizing system and in Deleuze and Guattari's ontology, difference is conceptualized beyond notions of replication, reproduction and representation. "In conceptualizing difference in and of itself, a difference which is not subordinated to identity, Deleuze and Guattari invoke notions of becoming and of multiplicities beyond the mere doubling or proliferation of singular, unified, subjectivities (Grosz, 1994, p. 164). I suggest that this notion of difference is where SPs in their irreducibility to a single identity reside; as exterior to the "Royal science" of the "State apparatus" and as forces unto themselves. "They are a war machine – an assemblage of multiplicities defined through their capacities to undergo permutations, transformations and realignments" (Grosz, 1994, 225). Rhizomatic in its non linear and heterogeneous connectivity, the work in which SPs engage especially in teaching settings is essentially generative and affirmative.

6.3 The war machine/nomads

> The primary determination of a nomad is to occupy and hold a smooth space: it is this aspect that determines them as a nomad (Deleuze & Guattari, 1987, p. 410).

Nomad science is characterized less by the absence of certainty than by an operative logic of movement and dynamic relationship between material forms and affective forces. The terms nomad/war machine/pragmatics/schizoanalyis are in relationship to each other as building material. Deleuze and Guattari construct an alternative praxis out of the relations between material and aesthetic forces that turn all notions of a direct and stable reality upside down. In this space of "between" and "becoming", examinations of metamorphosis, movement, acting, affect and the world of SPs takes on a different shape. Just as a royal science is tied to the concerns of "State" so too is a nomad science tied to the "war machine" through an elaborated system of thought, science, philosophy and action. "The war machine is the invention of the nomads (in so far as it is exterior to the state apparatus […]" (Deleuze & Guattari, 1987, p. 380).

SPs can be understood as the original war machine as defined by Deleuze and Guattari because they are exterior to the institutions and profession in which they are located and have been created through relationships of antagonism.

> Unlike the State – logos – which reproduces itself remaining identical to itself across its variations….The war machine's form of exteriority is such that it exists only in its own metamorphosis…in all flows and currents that only secondarily allow themselves to be appropriated by the State (1987, p. 360).

Unlike Foucault's notion of resistance the relationship between the state and the nomad war machine generates not only new subjectivities and knowledges within other discursive spaces: it produces "difference" that is transformative. The war machine effects new assemblages of desire along lines of becoming that can not be appropriated in their entirety by state apparatuses for measurement or repetition. In teaching sessions with SPs where bad news or grief are part of the scenario a medical trainee sitting with a crying person unable to fall back on clinical information to alleviate the situation is invaluable and immeasurable. "In every respect the war machine is of another species, another nature, another origin than the State apparatus" (Deleuze & Guattari, 1987, p. 352). It is singular and particular to a moment. This refers not only to the assemblages that are engendered through affect but also to SPs' physical, institutional and professional locations.

6.3.1 Nomad Space

> Nomad space is "smooth" or open ended. One can rise up at any point and move to any other. Its mode of distribution is *nomos*: arraying oneself in an open space (hold the street) (Massumi, 1987, p. xiii).

Movement is inherent, in all aspects of the history of the standardized patient program itself, as well as, to the lives and work of SPs in our particular program. Physically we have moved location nine times in our twenty-six year history and have never paid for space until our most recent incarnation. We have occupied space as nomads and itinerants relying on the generosity of those who value our contributions. In parallel with our physical transience we also inhabit the white spaces of the university's organizational structure – a vast ambiguous space in which we have thrived as outsiders to all departments and faculties who "use" us. As outsiders we have been able to develop work that is broader in scope and more inventive than could have been possible to imagine had we been tied to reporting structures of one sort or another. It is a disenfranchised freedom no other SP program can claim.

The U of T SPP is a large and thriving animal that looks like both a business and an academic entity. Our moves from one site to another have been as a result of our ever expanding size – from 30 or 40 SPs to over 500 – and the accompanying traffic, noise and activity, or because we no longer "fit" our host's mandate and needs for the space we occupy. We have never had a home *per se* or put down roots, and this transience informs our day to day engagement with each other and those with whom we work. It generates a resourcefulness (everything is possible) and affection for each other and our work, which is situated in desire - desire that produces realities. Physical and institutional space represents a strategic commitment, and requires us to maintain agility through informal and extrinsic relations. In other words invention and reinvention is part of our survival. Inhabiting a nomad space as an organization means that there is responsiveness to ideas that fly in from many different quarters and agility to move with them in unexpected ways which generate multiple possibilities.

Nomad space is qualitatively different. It is relational space rather than one confined by gravity, allowing for possibilities of movement of many kinds in many directions. The possibility of capitulating to the formation of the state apparatus in which stability and order override movement is always in tension with immanent relationships of the band or pack type. "Packs, bands are groups of the rhizome type, as opposed to the arborescent type that centres around organs of power" (Deleuze & Guattari, 1987, p.358). The distinction between rhizomatic movement and arborescent systems is central to Deleuze and Guattari's thesis, with arborescence aligned with reproduction, "tracing", and understood to be; "hierarchical systems with centers of significance and subjectification, central automata like organized memories" (1987, p. 16). Beyond regulations and rules there is a fertile connectivity which needs to remain central to our ethos. This singularity of movement which is prolific and non linear Deleuze refers to as mapping. Artists are much like academics in that we carry our resources within us - our tools go where we go. SPs rhizomatically territorialize along lines that join with other lines taking different paths. We also deterritorialize in innumerable ways, connecting and creating different machines through a plethora of interdisciplinary and inter-professional alliances. We are connected to the path not the destination, although we are not ignorant of the importance or value of established points or nodes along the way. This freedom of movement and independence makes us dangerous. In other words we are aware of and abide by the rules of the University but at this point live outside of its regulatory demands for accreditation and accountability. War machines are exterior to the State and enjoy a great deal of autonomy in relation to the State... "and answer to other rules... which animate a questioning of hierarchy [...]" (1987, p.358).

The creative, chaotic, generative, elements that make up a functioning field of practice, such as theatre, painting, music, once it is appropriated by institutional or state logos is reshaped with all the "dynamic nomadic notions such as becoming, heterogeneity, and infinitesimal passage to the limit, eliminated, and civil state and ordinal rules imposed upon it"

(Deleuze & Guattari, 1987, p. 363). The state needs to own and harness heterogeneity and becoming for its own ends. It does not have its own war machine and needs its energy in a different form in order "to move from one point to another, to prevent turbulence – to fall in line" (1987, 363). A different model, that of:

> nomad science and the war machine, on the other hand, consists in being distributed by turbulence across a smooth space, in producing a movement that holds space and simultaneously affects all of its points, instead of being held by space in a local movement from one specific point to another (Deleuze & Guattari, 1987, p. 363).

6.3.2 Nomad Professionals

> It would seem that a whole nomad science develops eccentrically, one that is very different from the royal or imperial sciences. Furthermore this nomad science is continually "barred" inhibited, or banned by the demands and conditions of the State science (Deleuze & Guattari, 1987, p. 362).

Within the field of human simulation the lure of legitimacy creates a strong pull toward conformity and alignments of one sort or another, either to a particular profession, academic location or definitive description of the work in which SPs engage. However I suggest that remaining as outsiders to medicine is necessary in order to retain the distinctive value that unscientific multiple perspectives offers. SPs within the health professions live at this intersection. There exists ongoing tension between territorializing with the health professions in ways that establish legitimacy and recognition, and deterritorializing as irreducible packs of becoming patients, always just outside the gates. This tension plays out in different fields of interaction. It is one thing to enact a patient story in such a way as to shatter preset notions about what a communication "should" look like, and another to impose a non scientific understanding into a scientific presentation or venue. The warrior[3] is both highly valued for what he can affect while always in danger of being an embarrassment to those who invite him in. "From the State perspective the originality of the man of war, his eccentricity, necessarily appears in a negative form: stupidity, deformity, madness, illegitimacy, usurpation, sin" (Deleuze & Guattari, 1987, p. 353-354).

Human simulation represents a nomad science not only in the actuality but in its conception. The ruling apparatus is invested in molar systems tied to repetition without difference, stable identity, and a linear and historical chronology of time and place, while the war machine is invested in a "non unitary subjectivity and a nomadic, dispersed, fragmented vision which is nonetheless functional and coherent and accountable mostly because it is embedded and embodied" (Braidotti, 2006, p. 4).

The variable and singular nature of SP/nomadic subjectivity is a contested space of mutations that pushes against the legislative and constituent primacy of royal science. "It is necessary to reach the point of conceiving of the war machine as itself a pure form of exteriority, whereas the state apparatus constitutes the form of interiority we habitually take as a model or according to which we are in the habit of thinking [...]" (Deleuze & Guattari, 1987, p. 354). The battle plays out within the professionalizing processes of the field of human simulation project which has grown internationally in and through its close proximity to a positivist medical science and its medical education paradigm. Its professional form: Association of Standardized Patient Educators, (ASPE) is a conscious mirror of the large medical educational associations with whom it is considered important to align for legitimacy. Ties with medical simulation and their royal society, The Society for Simulation in Health Care (SSIH), are tightening with debates over accreditation of simulation programs and certification of trainers occurring at high levels, internationally. Protection of standards and creation of best practices, are moves to "guard the gate" and "hold the fort" territorializing through replicating legitimacy and power according to State form. There is an antagonism set up. This new State apparatus requires a war machine and nomads, as it does not have its own. The artists and outsiders – the "not quite" and "never to be" legitimate, are still valued as important contributors however their value is contingent on their outsider status much like the warrior hired by the state. This is a work in progress with possibilities for subversion or attack by nomadic elements who are not committed to legitimacy through homogenizing and universalizing forces.

6.4   Becoming Patient

> Becoming is an intransitive process; it is not about becoming anything in particular (Braidotti, 2006, p. 163).

In this section I examine the becoming patient process in which SPs engage as a unique affective variation on the work of acting. Interlinking the two fields of practice while allowing each its singular profile, I am engaging in what Braidotti calls a "transposition: a creative leap that produces a prolific in-between space" (Braidotti, 2006, p. 5). Most closely aligned with theories of acting and notions of metamorphosis, I suggest that the process of training and portraying patient roles as a unique form of pedagogy for teaching medical students and practicing health professional is a distinct hybrid – a rhizomatic offshoot with elements that are exterior to both acting, and other forms of experiential learning.

Within this discussion I will examine notions of: itinerancy and processes of "following" as they relate to the discussion of simulation as a nomad/war machine, affect as a material force, and, assemblages of desire that shift ontologically the possibilities of an engaged praxis.

6.4.1 Mary Rice (child abuser)

This is the name of the role I was recruited to learn and portray for a self assessment research study for Family Practice Residents.[4] It was a pre/post research design in which the Family Practice Residents were to rank themselves regarding self perceived confidence and competence following an interview with a standardized patient. As such the project was aligned with medicine's neoliberal and modernist notions in which evaluation of individuals using the standardized patient performance as a dependent variable is part of a professional normalizing process. That I was a part of this exercise as a disruptive agent also fits with the outsider status of SPs. The role and my portrayal of it were intended to challenge both the skills of the clinician and their sense of efficacy as a family practitioner. As in an OSCE the performance of the candidate was rated by an observing clinician. Unlike in an OSCE, the candidate was also rated by me following which our ratings as "experts" were compared against the candidates' self report.

The first thing I remember about the role I was to portray is that I performed it a long time ago when my own kids were 5 and 8 years old. This is important in that they played a part in my process of "becoming child abuser". The other memory that stands out is the great number of times I performed this role during the initial project for which it was created and how each felt distinctly different from the others. This is not to say that it was a different role each time; to the contrary the facts of the case remained the same. What was distinct was a singularity created between us in each encounter. What kind of performance is this?

> One does not represent, one engenders and transverses (Deleuze & Guattari, 1987, p. 364).

6.4.2 Preparing for Mary

Mary is real to me. Her story and her life are imaginable and are therefore possible to inhabit. Like taking on any role I have to learn Mary's story: I am single mother, live on welfare. I used to work as a waitress but can't afford to anymore because I would lose my monthly support and probably wouldn't make enough money to be able to pay for my daughter, Melissa's child care. She is two years old and has tons of energy – she never stops. We just moved three months ago into a basement unit in boarding house in Parkdale. This is completely across town from where I used to live and I don't know anyone or the neighbour hood at all. It is noisy and scary from what I can tell. Melissa's father Doug has been out of the picture since just after she was born and good riddance. He is a drunk and is out of control sometimes so I don't want him around. He has never come to visit Melissa which is the way I want it. We used to drink together, wine or I used to… I can't afford it anymore… but I still have my smokes. I can't give those up; they are all I have to myself when I need a break and man do I need a break from this kid. Twenty-four hours a friggin' day with no other adult to talk to. I am losing my mind. I have no money but I have to get out of this room-and-a- half they call an apartment. We have cockroaches and silver fish. I don't know which is worse. So when we do get out Melissa wants everything she sees – candy, toys – sometimes I just take her into Zellers to look around and play with stuff but that doesn't always work out….So last night I was trying to get her to bed and she was crying about something, I don't even know what and …I lost it!! I didn't mean to hurt her but she would not shut up! I grabbed her by the arm and she fell and I then I threw her into her crib. She wouldn't stop crying and now she is holding her arm and I am swearing and crying and….Shit!!!

She cried all night long and I can't stand it. I feel so awful. I am afraid that I've really hurt her so I take her into the family medicine clinic at St. Joe's and tell them that she fell off the bed and hurt her arm. They x-rayed her arm. It was broken! And, put it in a cast and now I just want to take her home I feel so bad I can't believe I did that. I just want to get out of here but they want to talk to me first. Shit!

I can feel the hopelessness as I write this out: The sadness at the core of this woman's existence. She loves her daughter and Melissa is by all accounts a cherubic kid. From my understanding and experience of Mary what is going on has nothing to do with the kind of person she is – a "child abuse" – but a whole complex of hopes and frustrations and hellish reality from which she can not escape. This is who I need to inhabit: Someone at the end of hope.

It is a long walk up to embodying this role. I have two little boys, and am in no way in Mary's circumstances. What I have to do is *more* than imagine for myself the possibility that I would act in the same way as Mary. I need to deterritorialize, taking a line away from myself in order to inhabit those places where I do want to scream and throw and lose it with my own kids while holding on to the piece of me that knows that as much as I could - I wouldn't and don't. I create a possibility for myself of going over the edge so that I am not acting. It is a tricky walk both physically and emotionally and it takes time. In this process, "engagement with linear historical time and place are different from the discontinuous time of becoming" (Braidotti, 2005, p.155). .The story itself is embedded in the dismantling of a self; becoming a Body Without Organs (BwO)[5] and an emptying out the self, opening it out to possible encounters with an unknown outside.

It is an act of "following". "From the point of view of nomad science which presents itself as an art as much as a technique…it *follows* the connections between singularities of matter and the traits of expression and lodges on the level of these connections whether they be natural or forced" (Deleuze & Guattari, 1987, p. 369). "Following is different from the ideal of reproduction. Not better just different" (p. 372). The art of following is what distinguishes the standardized performances that reproduce schizophrenia symptoms from a singular event. "One is obligated to follow when one is in search of the 'singularities' of a matter or rather of a material and not out to discover form….when one engages in a continuous variation of variables instead of extracting constants from them etc" (1987, p. 372). Referring to this as an ambulant model of science Deleuze goes onto say that.

> And the meaning of Earth completely changes: with the legal model [of reproduction], one is constantly reterritorializing around a point of view, on a domain, according to a set of constant relations; but with the ambulant model, the process of deterritorialization

> constitutes and extends the territory itself (Deleuze & Guattari, 1987, p. 372).

The various exchanges that I as Mary will have with the health professionals will be singular and embody the risk of moving in unknown territory, in spite of what we think or think we know when we encounter each other in the room. There is a building and mapping process and a shattering of everything that is coherent or whole about what I have built. Mary's life is of a different speed and intensity. "This movement takes place on a "plane of consistency which is the intersection of all concrete forms" (Deleuze & Guattari, 1987, p. 251). A plane of consistency refers to a fixed plane that has nothing to do with form or a figure or a design or a function. It eschews interiority or the ground of deep meaning for the surface. It is "a fixed plane upon which things are distinguished from one another only by speed and slowness. What we are talking about is not the unity of substance but the infinity of the modifications that are part of one another on this unique plane of life" (1987, p. 254).

> In short, between substantial forms and determined subjects, *between the two,* there is not only a whole operation of demonic local transports but a natural play of haecceities, degrees, intensities, events, and, accidents that compose individuations totally different from those of the well formed subjects that receive them (Deleuze & Guattari, 1987, p. 253).

It is here that acting as a metamorphosis – a becoming other - along dimensions of intensity, slowness and speeds comes forward. It is not imitation or mimesis but rather a process in which you "…make your organism enter into composition with *something else* in such a way that the particles emitted from the aggregate thus composed will be integrally [other] as a function of the relation of movement and rest…" (1987, p. 274). Deleuze describes a becoming animal process in which: "Robert De Niro walks "like" a crab in a certain film sequence; but, he says, it is not a question of his imitating a crab; it is a matter of making something that has to do with crab enter into composition with the image, with the speed of the image" (Deleuze & Guattari, 1987, p. 274). It is beyond reason or thought it is sensorial. There is both an "in between" and a "more than" in the taking on of Mary that exceeds the space of reproduction. This entails a nomad trajectory into indefinite, unknown territory that must be inhabited in the present moment of exchange.

6.4.3 Enacting Mary

> Feelings become uprooted from the interiority of the subject to be projected violently outward into a milieu of pure exteriority that lends them an incredible velocity, a capturing force: love or hate, they are no longer feelings but affects (Deleuze & Guattari, 1987, p. 356).

As Mary, I spoke with over fifty health professionals in the space of a couple of months. Each one was given the same information before entering the room to speak with me about Melissa. They were given a task and the following information.

> You are about to see Mary Rice, the mother of 2 year old Melissa.
>
> Mary brought Melissa up to the Family Medicine department stating her daughter had been playing on the bed the night before and had fallen off. Mary decided to bring Melissa to the Family Medicine Department this morning because she wouldn't stop crying and was holding her arm.
>
> You examined Melissa earlier and x-rayed her arm. Melissa appeared neglected. The radiologist stated the x-ray showed a metaphyseal fracture suggestive of abuse.
>
> You must meet with the mother again, discuss your concerns, and indicate legally you must inform the Children's Aid Society. Melissa is in the fracture room getting a cast on. She is fine.
>
> You have 10 minutes.

When the Resident walks in I feel his contempt and disapproval tinged with something else less discernible rush into the room in a wave. I am not prepared for this as Mary or as Nancy. White coat, clipboard with notes, not looking at me directly, he sits down beside the desk.

After asking me if I am Melissa's mother he begins to tell me that Melissa has broken her arm and is now with a nurse who is taking care of her while she is having a cast put on. In response to my shock over the fact that she has broken he arm, he proceeds to tell me that the x-ray reveals a metaphyseal fracture. *Huh?* Pause....I don't like this cool calm man in white using big words about my little girl and implying secret knowledge of my life. I ask when I can see Melissa and take her home. He suggests that she may have to stay in the hospital for a few days. *"For a fracture?"* I don't believe him. *"Well where is she I need to see her? She's never been away from me for more than a couple of hours."* My blood is rising. The doctor asks "Why don't you tell me what happened last night" *"Why? She fell off the bed and I guess broke her arm. She's a busy kid. All kids break something at some point right?" "I should have brought her in last night but I didn't think it was that bad until this morning."* Pause. He asks, "Do you live alone with Melissa?" *"Why? What does that have to do with anything?"* He continues "Do you have a boyfriend?" *"That is none of your business."* Looking at his clipboard he asks "Do you smoke?" "Drink alcohol?" Do street drugs?" There is a stream of questions and I sit stunned. *"Let me see my kid."* Doctor: "Is she in day care?" *No I can't afford it"* Doctor: "What do you do when you get angry with Melissa?" *What do you mean? I do what all parents do. I yell some I give her a time out. Like that."* Do you have any family or support system to help you? Her father? *"No".*

The inquisition continues – a fact finding, clue following attempt to get at the "truth" of the situation, ultimate success achieved in getting a confession out of me. I am caught between despair and rage and not breathing. He's not listening or can't hear any of my responses and I am intensely angry, vibrating in my bones, at his dismissive contempt and identification of me as a "type" – the irresponsible and negligent mother on welfare. Finally he tells me his secret. "We know that Melissa's injury was not caused by a fall but by someone pulling her arm and I am wondering if someone other than you could have done this? *"What are you saying? Are you accusing me of breaking Melissa's arm on purpose? Are you?"* Doctor: "The x-ray is conclusive about the kind of break she has suffered." *"Well then your x-ray is wrong."* I am not going to share anything with this man. *"I am taking Melissa home now."* I get ready to leave the office. I see him look at me anxiously and he says, "I am sorry I am going to have to call the Children's Aid Society… Melissa will have to stay…" *"What?" The Children's Aid Society." "Who the fuck do you think you are sitting over there so fucking sure of yourself and your facts? Fuck off and let me have my child." You can't keep her here."* Pause. My chest is tight and I can sense that the resident is shocked, like I physically hit him, which is what it felt like to me. Is there hope of any kind is what I am thinking. *"They are going to take Melissa away from me."* He responds in a very cool tone "It is my responsibility to protect Melissa and make sure that she doesn't get hurt further."

We are now on opposite sides of a very large chasm. I am the enemy to be thwarted as part of his holy duty to society. This resident has confirmed his decision about me in this interaction that I am "the abuser" and all that such a constellation of behaviours entails according to facts that he has been taught. I am white trash who smokes and drinks away the welfare cheque while neglecting and abusing my child. *"What do you know about living on no money in a cockroach infested apartment?"* He responds "Are you Catholic or Protestant?" *"What?"* I am speechless. He says from far away. "I have to call the Children's Aid society and have them set up a home visit. There are two organizations in Toronto…" He cannot see me or hear me. *"Oh my God. They can't come to my hole of an apartment they will take her away for sure."* He says "I am sorry but that may be the best for Melissa and they won't take her away unless it is absolutely necessary. They try to keep families together not tear them apart". I am silent, and lost and hopeless. There is nothing I can say or do. It is over. What remains? There remain bodies which are forces, nothing but forces [….]" (Deleuze, 1989, p. 139).

203

This is a heart aching exchange in which there is little understanding arrived at despite all of the questions. We both feel stunned. Affects do things – create "becomings", unhooking us from taken for granted understandings, identities and knowledges. "They can sum up a set of disparate circumstances in a shattering blow" (Massumi, 1987, p. xi). Unpacking this exchange is not about communication skills or even "active listening skills" that may have provided him with the tools to engage me "empathically." This exchange seeps much deeper into the seams of our social and cultural fabric and the professional interpretations about what it means to be a "good doctor". In this exchange, the rigid segmentarity of royal science's molar or gridded lines are intertwined with many molecular lines of becoming, one of the most apparent of which has to do with human suffering –which the practice of medicine is charged with, if not ameliorating, at very least acknowledging.

Affect is captured and emotions coded and over coded, according to medicine's disciplinary and juridical notions of professional responsibility. It overflows from that of doctor and patient to that of" becoming–doctor" and "becoming–patient" as enacted in this exchange. But the regime of the war machine is on the contrary that of affects, which relate only to the moving body in itself, to speeds (intensities) and compositions of speed among elements…. It is a movement of decoding of another sort, where there is no longer any goal: attacks, counterattacks and headlong plunges" (Deleuze & Guattari, 1987, p. 400). There are implications here for the ways in which suffering can be potentially recognized, acknowledged and addressed. Nowhere in the exchange between myself and the junior doctor is there any recognition of Mary's suffering related to her life situation and her present social or economic circumstances. She is a dilemma to be solved, guilty party, perpetrator, with the victim already assigned before we begin our dance. As such Mary is turned into a problem.

6.4.3.1 Surfaces of Skin, Action and Gesture

Because our exchange was part of a research project, the resident and I were not allowed to have a conversation about our experiences. Mary however has had many incarnations in teaching settings and the unpacking of an exchange always involves holding space for the creative edge of possibility. Walking away with molecules rearranged.

My starting point in taking this event apart with a medical trainee is that teaching is an embodied cultural and political undertaking that shapes and is shaped by emotion and affect. There is a line of flight that a trainee, and I and an observing physician could follow in our mutual exploration after the exchange is over. Vocabulary for such a conversation is emergent. What happened? How did he put his picture of me together? What informed this picture? What is left out? What didn't he hear me say? What did I not hear him say? These are not clinical questions nor are they addressing skills, or abilities as residing inside either one of us.

Taking up Sarah Ahmed's work on emotion as political and cultural work I am interested in interrogating the ways in which emotions shape ideas and enactments and get projected onto bodies – some bodies but not others. For Ahmed, emotions are experienced in the body as mediated by history and are part of a cultural politics. As she states: "The 'truths' of this world are dependent on emotions, on how they move subjects and stick them together" (Ahmed, 2004, p. 170). Her analysis of my exchange with the resident might focus on the ways in which our affective exchange involved:

> [..] a reading of the world and a reading of the reading, dependent on past interpretations that were not necessarily made by us but that come before us and that we brought to this particular instance, where feelings did not reside in subjects or objects but were produced as effects of circulation (2004, p. 8).

It is a historical and political undertaking placing us both within a larger social context, mediated through our embodied exchange. My exchange with the resident trainee is also an event held in space and time between us which in its immanence brings me back to Deleuze and Guattari and nomadic following. Actors and SPs are nomadic, bringing to their work skills related to their itinerancy and the primacy of holding the open space of possibility.

> The nomad knows how to wait; he has infinite patience... distribut[ing] himself in a smooth space (in the space of possibility): he occupies, inhabits and holds that space. That is his territorial principle (Deleuze & Guattari, 1987, p.381).

In the act of following there are no prescribed answers to unpack. Ahmed speaks about a "space of wonder" where outcomes are held back in order to keep open the possibility of discovery. This is the liminal edge of a pedagogy in which bodies actively engage in emotional and affective work. Such an approach creates a space for discovery and the development of ethics through an aesthetics of wonder. "The capacity for wonder is the space of opening up to the surprise of each combination; each body, which turns this way or that, impresses upon others, affecting what they can do. Wonder keeps bodies and spaces open to the surprise of others" (2004, p.183).

6.5 Assemblages of Desire: SP-Actor-Nomad

A pedagogy of desire as outlined by Zembylas (2007) takes Deleuze and Guattari's theorization of desire from *a thousand plateaus* into the classroom "reclaiming desire as a legitimate *affective* and *relational practice"* (2007, p. 334). It is not bound to any set of "best teaching practices" or "appropriate methods" or "outcomes" but is a specific assemblage of transgressive, creative and pleasurable forces. Affect, emotion and desire are particular to a configuration in the moment. These assemblages take into account and disturb not only what story is going to be engaged and how but also all the contexts and experiences that different parties bring in fragments and pieces to the situation. Medical education settings create unique assemblages just as theatre and film form unique machines through assemblages of a different sort, with actors "becoming-other" in parallel but not identical processes to the "becoming other" of SPs.

There is a different assemblage created for an SP as "tool" or "weapon" when engaged in educational and assessment activities. An SP's directionality of focus shifts relationships in slightly but not entirely different ways in each of these assemblages. It is different again from an actor enacting a complex story for an audience night after night, or frozen in time on screen. There is no single term that can define it. It is a difference in assemblage – in pack allegiances, same animal different type. Even in their most subversive affective activity SPs are always territorialized to the royal science of the health professions with an understanding that they would not exist except for this relationship. Actors territorialize along different lines with different relations of formation and deformation, producing audiences and spectacles at intensities distinct from those of SPs.

SPs may be seen to represent a simulacrum or copy of the real which comes to stand in for, and replace the real itself. Hayles (1993) suggests that "we are in the midst of a shift into virtual reality (a disembodied and disaffected space) where language, information and subjectivity are never 'really' present in themselves" (cited in Boler, 1996, p. 13). Joan Scott (1992) critiques the idea that experience is direct evidence. She suggests a more complex relationship between the "real" of experience as a transparent rendering of an event and the importance of showing how experience itself is constructed and not self evident or beyond scrutiny as a source of evidence. What is the nature of the gap that leaves in question an unproblematized relationship between the "real" and the acted? What is at stake here is an understanding about the experience of "real" suffering on the part of the people enacting different patient stories whether they are acting or not. Are SPs, similar to what Spelman (1997) describes as "spiritual bellhops", that is carriers of experience from which others can benefit? (cited in Diedrich, 2007, p. 105). Is this investment essentially different from that of actors performing a role? They are in the same constitutive relationship to their work as actors. Some suggest that the value of engaging SPs to perform illness narratives is that they are not "real" in that the actor doesn't actually suffer the condition being performed. Others suggest that such encounters are "real" for being able to evoke genuine responses in the interviewee. Irony prevails when a SP is enacting a role of a suffering patient who has access to support and resources that they in their "real" situation do not (Taylor, 2011).

Both actors and SPs affectively embody complex social and cultural stories at the limit of certainty. There is a network of lines and intersections that cross between the controllable and the knowable and that which remains mysterious and uncertain. SPs work at several of these intersections; between ideas about and practices related to illness and health, visible symptoms and expressions, procedures and practices of amelioration and the affects that disrupt the stability of such combinations. We ask unanswerable questions from a realm beyond medicine inviting health professionals to join in a "wordless not knowing" or what Lisa Deidrich (2007) identifies as a "practicing at a loss" (p. 157) and an "ethics of failure" (p. xxi). It is an active witnessing. Both actors and SPs are war machines of a different sort. "An ideological, artistic or scientific movement can be a potential war machine, to the precise extent to which it draws in relation to a plane of consistency, a creative line of flight, a smooth space of displacement" (Deleuze & Guattari, 1987, p. 423).

6.6 Conclusion

> On the side of the nomadic assemblages and war machines, it is a kind of rhizome with its gaps, detours, subterranean passages and stems, openings, traits and holes etc. On the other side, the sedentary assemblages and State apparatuses effect a capture…put the traits of expression into a form or code, make the holes resonate together, plug the lines of flight, subordinate the technological operations to the work model, impose upon the connections a whole regime of arborescent conjunctions." (Deleuze & Guattari, 1987, p. 415).

Where do SPs stand in this configuration? A Deleuzian perspective on affect and emotion as it relates to the work of SPs expands our ability to imagine differently the ways in which bodies and desire are configured in processes of becoming "other". "The life of the nomad is the intermezzo. Even the elements of his dwelling are conceived in terms of the trajectory that is forever mobilizing them" (Deleuze & Guattari, 1987, p. 380). Transposed always "between" and at the edge of creative possibility, the nomad war machine is always moving. SPs are vectors of deterritorialization – in other words a medium through which transformational learning and new understanding is created.

Multiple possibilities collide when critically examining implications of enacting clinical reality from the lay person's perspective. Performances of empathy and compassion by a health care trainee which are often reduced to a demonstration of skills and abilities for "dealing" with variations of "the difficult patient", such as the "harried housewife", the "pregnant lesbian", "the angry patient", become an affective charge doubling back on itself. The shared embodied experiences are a liminal space at the threshold of medical cultures' inside and outside. Borderlands that traditionally exist as sites of contestation, risk and risk taking, render the liminal performers vulnerable. Playing with prescribed representational ideas about medical student, clinician teacher, patient and standardized patient performances opens a space for questions while not abandoning responsibility and accountability as central to the relationships enacted. Indeterminacy and uncertainty introduced in this way are the purview of the nomad war machine. "The point of nomad subjectivity is to identify a line of flight….a creative alternative space of becoming that would fall not between the mobile and immobile, the resident and the foreigner, but within these categories" (Braidotti, 2006, p. 60). This approach includes border crossings and non-unitary identities that emphasize the complexity and the relationality of affect for all parties.

In this chapter I have engaged a rhizomatic method of analysis outlining an alternative reading of the relations and forces shaping the professional work and location of standardized patients within medical education. Employing Deleuze and Guattari's treatise on nomadology and the war machine SPs are figured as outsiders to the profession and educational field in which they are engaged. From this location SPs are able to make unique contributions both in unsettling taken for granted truths and in embodying an affective ethics creating space for imagining differently what t means to be in relation to suffering.

Notes

1. The following checklist is a generic example of OSCE checklists that are used for examination purposes. Actual OSCE checklists are secure and are not available for reproduction as they represent exam answers. There is large amount of financial and professional time invested in the creation of checklists specific to different levels of student, diagnosis and exam purpose, for example and final year exam vs. a licensing exam. The example below is meant to provide the reader with a sense of the structure of such checklists with the binary yes/no or in some cases done/ not done classification that direct the training and possible responses of the SP.

History   **Yes/No**

Asks questions regarding

    Duration of symptoms

    Location

    Radiation

    Quality of pain

    Exacerbating factors

    Relieving factors

    Nausea/vomiting

    Fever/chills

    Previous history of symptoms

    Asks about appetite

    History of hematemesis

    History of melena

    Last bowel movement

>   Alcohol use, must quantify
>
>   Medications
>
> **Physical**
>
>   Appropriate draping and exposure
>
>   Inquires re location of maximal discomfort
>
>   Inspects for masses, discoloration distension, asymmetry
>
>   Auscultates before palpating
>
>   Assesses
>
>   Palpates abdomen lightly all four quadrants
>
>   Palpates more deeply all four quadrants
>
>   Notes presence of guarding or rigidity
>
>   Checks for rebound tenderness
>
>   In all manoeuvres observes patient for distress

2. In the United States there are traditionally no physicians in the exam rooms during SP examinations. SPs complete computerized checklists after the end of each encounter. Physicians may watch from a centralized computer room in order to check on both the accuracy of the SP portrayal and their checklist completion. This configuration fundamentally changes the work and the roles in which SPs engage in examination settings. Much more time and money is spent on training SPs for accurate checklist completion and recall strategies while cases themselves are simplified in order to achieve a high level of reliability rather than relational reality.

3. Deleuze and Guattari are critiqued by feminists for the masculinist essentialism of many of their concepts. Referencing "warrior" as masculine in this passage is another example of the ways in which

language has material implications. Like their idea of "becoming woman" as a stage through which one passes before "becoming imperceptible" gendering concepts like warrior and woman excludes individuals from particular locations within their apparatus of desire as power. I am hoping that my analysis troubles this exclusion, recognizing women as inhabiting this location as productively if not as visibly as men.

4. Martin D., Regehr G., Hodges B., McNaughton N. Using Videotaped Benchmarks to Improve Self Assessment Ability of family Practice Residents. *Academic Medicine*, Vol. 73, No 11/November1998. 1201-1206. Of interest for me is the erasure of Mary's story in this article which identifies it only as one of the tools used to measure the residents self assessment performance.

5. A Body without organs or BwO refers to Artaud's passage in *To Have Done with the Judgment of God.* (1982, *Antonin Artaud: Four texts.* Transl. Clayton Eshleman and Norman Glass. Los Angeles. Panjandrum. In which he states; "For tie me down if you want to / but there is nothing more useless than an organ. // When you have given him a body without organs, / then you will have delivered him from all of his automatisms and /restored him to his true liberty. (p. 79)". Deleuze and Guattari state; "The BwO is what remains when you take everything away. (151)" It can be occupied or populated only by intensities. (153) It is "the unformed, unorganized, nonstratified, or destratified body and all its flows: subatomic and submolecular particles, pure intensities, prevital and prephysical free singularities. (157-58)". "The BwO is desire; it is that which one desires and by which one desires" (165). It is a force.

Chapter 7 A Deleuzian Enactment of a Foucauldian Space

7.0   Introduction

In this chapter I theorize a particular performance of nomadology in which affect and emotion are central political media. The event that I will be describing was staged as part of a conference entitled "Performing the World" in which performing artists, community organizers, theatre workers, educators, scholars, youth workers, students, social workers, psychotherapists, psychologists, medical doctors, health workers, and business executives from thirty one countries participated in discussions and performances in answer to the question; Can performance change the world? For my colleague[1] and me it was an invitation to participate in a decentring of affiliations and ideas about medicine and patients and standardized patients through an enactment of the medical educational gaze. In other words we wanted to create an event in which the audience had an opportunity to feel assembled as medical trainees according to particular taken for granted professional expectations. It was political because we aspired to evoke the felt effects of power in both a collective as well as individual sense.

7.1   Performance and Pedagogy

There are innumerable ways in which performance and theatre are employed critically for education. Raising awareness of inequities through observing and reflecting on performances is one way. Taking part in improvised and scripted role plays that address social, political and economic inequities is another (Theatre of the Oppressed, Forum Theatre, 1979). As a form of performance, human simulation falls ambiguously in between these two and in between demonstration and theatre. It has the possibility of acting as a critical challenge to think and act differently; to embody situated material effects of power from a different location.

In the open-ended space of learning through interaction the ethical is cultural, political and economic, engendering effects that, are as Braidotti describes it, both "embodied and embedded" in specific social networks. Performance pedagogy entails embodied experiences in which it is possible to recognize socio-historical contexts as integral for collaborative learning. In other words it is situated learning. As a forum for thinking and acting differently together it offers opportunities to experience learning aesthetically and affectively. Learning that intersects with theory in this way is activated as an ethical practice. Ethics as a situated practice invites different perspectives to collide and for desire and discomfort to instigate questioning that removes morality as a stable property of individuals. Such decentering strips "should" from relational engagements and bans "appropriate" to the garbage dump of no longer needed or useful weapons.

> Performance is always a doing and a thing done: on the one hand "embodied acts in specific sites, witnessed by others (and/or the watching self)," while on the other, the completed event framed in time and space and remembered, misremembered, interpreted and passionately revisited across a pre-existing discursive field (Elin Diamond, 1996, p.1).

Learning through performance (not only simulation) that is immediate and felt is also subject to epistemological frameworks that define and shape what is considered legitimate knowledge and pedagogy. It is an ethical project that hopes to expand the understandings of a dominant centre through activities that invite a "becoming other" through affective engagement. Following Braidiotti, I favour a radical ethics of transformation that shifts the focus from unitary to nomadic subjectivity and which "proposes an enlarged sense of interconnection between self and others, including the non human or "earth" others, by removing the obstacle of self centred individualism" (Braidotti, 2006, p. 35).

7.2   Performing the Medical Educational Gaze

Performance remakes and unmakes mimesis (Roach, 2010, p. 457).

7.2.1 Abstract

The following description was published in the "Performing the World" conference program.

> In our demonstration participants will be complicit in the process of constructing the "medical gaze" through their performance as trainees and clinicians receiving didactic teaching and demonstrations of various disease states and communication practices. Audience members will be asked to assess "student" performance, comment on observations and volunteer to interview "the difficult" patient. Reflective exercises and discussion will be engaged to deconstruct our collective learning experience.
>
> This presentation explores the ways in which privileged perspectives inherent in a western "medical gaze" and scientific method intersect with conceptions of illness/disease states and practitioner-patient relationships erasing the perspective of actual patients. Repeated and consistently honed "performances" of medical expertise reinforce hierarchical "roles" and evidence based practices that have little to do with health or patient experience.

7.2.2 Ethics Performed

The particular performance I am describing was a political practice of situated and shifting locations. As a form of philosophical nomadism the layered enactment in which my colleague and I engaged was an attempt to "address in both a critical and creative manner the role of the former centre in redefining power relations. Margins and centre shift and destabilize each other in parallel albeit asymmetrical movements" (Braidotti, 2006, p. 69). In the following description I am thinking about how enactments can be engaged as a way of embedding critical practice in specific, situated perspectives while avoiding universalistic generalizations or over arching master categories.

7.3 The Performance

7.3.1 Setting

We are in a smallish studio with white, bare walls. A projection screen is lowered at the front of the room. Off to the side is a rectangular table on which we place our props: a white lab coat, stethoscope, reflex hammer, clipboard with notes, checklists, handouts, scarf, small black notebook and pen, stop watch, bell, and whistle.

We arrange eighteen or so chairs into a teaching circle and place a syllabus on each. Two chairs are placed at the front of the room

7.3.2 Scene I

As audience file in we are seated and reading from the syllabus.

N: (*stands and reads aloud*) Affect and behaviour. Hyper arousal cluster...elated, over-excited, aggressive, unrealistically optimistic. (*sits*)

L: (*stands and reads aloud*) Vegetative cluster. Sluggish, stares into space, stays in bed, stays in room. (*sits*)

N: (*stands and reads aloud*) You should display proficiency at communicating and interacting appropriately with patients, families, health care personnel, and your peers. (*sits*)

L: (*stands and reads aloud*) Communication tools: normalizing, negotiating, legitimizing, repeating. (*sits*)

A handful of people file in and take seats. When most of the eighteen seats are filled and people are settled Nancy and LJ move to the props table. Nancy puts on the lab coat, with stethoscope and reflex hammer in the

pocket and picks up clipboard. LJ puts scarf in her hair and picks up the small notebook and pen and returns to her seat and bows her head in a SP freeze mode.

N/ Doctor: (*standing in front of the group*)

Welcome to the first day of your medical interviewing course. You will find that the syllabus on your chairs is full of helpful information. Look at the first page in particular entitled "Standards of Professional Behaviour for Medical Undergraduate and Postgraduate Students." It outlines the objectives and methods of assessment for professional and ethical performance by medical trainee in the Faculty of Medicine."

The package is a mock up of a student guide with all identifiers removed. The first page invokes the Oath of Hippocrates and outlines eight principles of behaviour that students are required to demonstrate, including the following statement. "Behaviour inconsistent with being a physician is viewed as a demonstration of lack of suitability to be a physician." The page ends with: "Breach of any of the above principles of behaviour may be cause for dismissal from a course or a program or failure to promote."

Such generalized proclamations about standards of behaviour and consequences for failure do a double service of identifying medicine as a privileged and sacred location while also threatening new comers to "act" as if they are physicians while not really knowing what this means. The information in the orientation manual effectively places medical training within a performance paradigm supporting notions of ethics as a demonstration of values ("demonstrate empathy and compassion for patients and families") reflecting an individualized moral imperative as part of its professional identity.

N/ Doctor: Today is "Difficult Patient Day". We will be working with a standardized patient to give you some practice managing difficult behaviours and learning how to gather precise and accurate information no matter what behaviour you face. Has anyone worked with Standardized Patients before? *(pause)* They're good actors, you'll enjoy it. You can't hurt them because they are not real and so it is very safe.

As you may know part of your mark in this course includes participation, so you will be expected to volunteer to do an interview; if not in this class than at some point in the next few weeks. It's expected that everyone will have a chance during the course to do two interviews and observe the others. I say again, your involvement will be an important part of your mark. If you are not the one in the hot seat we'll be asking you for feedback on what you see occurring in the different interviews. Your final mark will comprise of a written exam, a performance assessment, a clinical case report, a ward mark based on observations by your preceptors, and your reflections. Self-reflections will be assigned weekly. You're expected to complete 8 for the 12 week course. *(Silence)*

OK, so what is a difficult patient? What does it mean? Does it mean?

> The Non-compliant patient
>
> The talkative patient or over-inclusive patients
>
> The patient who's worried about everything
>
> What about emotions?

What can we do when patients yell, or when they cry?

Anyone here started a practicum? (*The audience members are subjected as first year students and so as the teacher I would know that none of the students would have experienced patient care as a medical trainee*). Had any contact with patients yet?

What are some of the challenges you might expect from this kind of patient?

One young woman put up her hand and answers that she thinks she might be labelled as a difficult patient herself as she has trouble with the western allopathic medical model. In our discussion following the performance she spoke about how frustrated and trapped she had felt at being subjected in this event to the role of the medical student.

N/ Doctor: What do you do that you think is difficult?

A: I don't know. I argue I guess.

N/ Doctor: Do you yell? Cry? Storm out? Are you non-compliant?

A: I sometimes don't agree with the way that I am treated as a patient and a woman. I sometimes feel talked down to and dismissed.

N/ Doctor: What do you do in these situations? I don't mean to badger you but you may encounter the challenges that you identify in your own behaviour, as the very difficulties you encounter in your future practice. How would you as a physician deal with you the difficult patient?

A: (silence)

Dr. N. hands out: the Interview Template, Observation Guide, and a Checklist[2]. The participants are now awash in paper. One fellow coming in late is visibly overwhelmed as he tries to make sense of all the different handouts.

N/ Doctor: *(Addressing the later comer)* You. What is your name?

B: *(says his name and sits down).*

N/ Doctor: Please do not be late again. It shows a lack of professionalism and you will be docked marks. We don't have a lot of time to get through everything that we need to. *(referring to the handouts)* These are the templates that you'll be working with today. Of course, you don't have to follow them too strictly but these are the areas that need to be covered in an interview. Are there any questions?

I briefly review the three new handouts. The first is "The Observation Guide" which breaks communication into three over arching categories: "Techniques" which is described as the tools or "what you use" to conduct an interview such as, bridging, clarifying, summarizing etc. The next category is "Styles" described as "How you do It": and the third is "Attitudes" described as "'Who you are': informed by values, beliefs, culture and environment." and includes within it "Being empathic", Being Honest", and "Having self awareness"

The document[3] created by the University of Toronto SPP for the purposes of teaching about communication skills is rife with jargon and works as both a heuristic device consequently elevating the professional status of the SPs using it. As non-clinician educators the document adopts medical educational terminology in such a way as to align the user with the medical profession as experts in the domain of communication. The document reifies communication processes and "therapeutic relationship" as skills to be acquired and honed through practice. Under theorized and generalized as a template for professional communication success, the document reflects an Emotional Intelligence and cognitive behavioural model of learning.

Like wise the checklist handout breaks down and isolates the content of an interview into discreet pieces. An example of checklist items for bipolar mania:

	correct not correct	
Asks about racing thoughts		1
Asks about spending		1
Asks about libido		1
Explores delusional religious ideation		1
Asks about suicidal ideation		1
Asks about homicidal ideation		1
Asks about hallucinations		1

Organization of the checklist into correct/not correct tasks represents an instrumental orientation to the encounter. It is another area of expertise for the SPs as mentioned in the earlier chapter regarding their ability to answer only what is asked and no more. There is also a widely adopted "process" checklist[3] (see notes at end of chapter) which organizes skills related to the "soft" or non clinical content of the interaction on a five point Likert scale. Included in the grid are: empathy, rapport, verbal and non verbal skills and coherence of the interview. For stations involving representations of mental illness these grids and accompanying measurement practices are potentially detrimental, rewarding heuristic and reductive thinking and practice.

The interview template is likewise a list of categories by which medical trainees learn to organize their conversations. Chief Complaint (CC), History of Present Illness (HPI), Review of Systems (ROS) etc. These acronyms represent important threshold markers of membership. SPs working in medical education are part of the privileged group who know what they mean and are required to reference them in their work. The categories become an organizational rubric for learning a role further privileging the special knowledge necessary to clinicians and required in the work of being an SP.

N/ Doctor: Good then we'll start with a demo. I will conduct an interview with our standardized patient who is playing the part of Janet Helen Cross (JHC) a patient with bipolar disorder. I believe that you had a PBL (problem based learning) session on this last week. I would like you to observe and use the templates that I have just handed out in order to comment on what I am doing with the patient. I am going to be calling "time outs" when I want to stop the action at which point we can talk about the exchange. Our SP will go back into freeze mode at these times.

The role of Janet Helen Cross is a case of Lithium overdose that was created for the Educating Future Physicians of Ontario (EFPO) project in the early 1990"s. It was created from an actual patient story and was originally trained in partnership with the psychiatrist author. It has become a staple for teaching and assessment and has been portrayed many times by many SPs over the years. Interestingly for this case, as for all of the cases which SPs enact, we have never had contact with the patient on whom the case was modelled or with any other patients who suffer from this disorder. Our understanding about the various manifestations and symptoms are only from the physicians' side of the creation.

The interview is to start and stop in the way mentioned above. L. has put a scarf in her hair and is writing intensely in a little black book that she had in her pocket

N/ Doctor: Ms. Cross what has brought you into the emergency room today?

L/JHC: *(writing in her notebook)* I have to get my prescription of lithium refilled today. It is very important. It is the seventh day of the seventh day and I can't waste time here talking to you.

N/ Doctor: Lithium. What are you prescribed lithium for?

L/JHC: *(on her feet and moving around the room)* I have a very important mission that involves travel. I have to go and tell the world about what is happening. Where did you get your earrings they match your eyes? There is a conspiracy and you are…

N/ Doctor (*interrupting*) May I call you Janet?

L/JHC: Yes. I am the second coming so my name is really like Jesus' name. People call me Janet but that's not my name anymore

N/ Doctor: (*slightly irritated*) Janet can you sit down for me? I see that you are very agitated right now. Can you sit down…please?

L/JHC: (comes and sits down) I have to go and tell the world about what is going on and finish my book. (stands up and starts moving again)

N/ Doctor: Time –out (*L sits down and continues writing disengaged from my conversation with the audience.*)

N/Doctor: What are you observing?

A number of the audience point out restlessness, fast speech, jumping from one topic to the other.

N/Doctor: What makes this a difficult patient?

Again audience members respond regarding the patients difficulty in finishing a thought or answering a question directly.

N/Doctor: Good. I am going to go back in. What would you like to know about Janet Helen Cross?

One audience member suggests: "More about her conspiracy theory?" Another asks "What is she on lithium for?" And another one "How much lithium?"

NANCY/Doctor: Good. Time–In

*L/JHC *(stands up).* Jesus H. Christ. Janet Helen Cross. See? *(as L stands up to show me her diagram I take her paper and pencil and she takes my clipboard.* **N/Doctor**: Yes I see Janet (*I give her my lab coat, stethoscope and reflex hammer and she gives me her scarf and little black book and pencil)*

(* signifies a change of roles)

N/JHC: See? I knew I was special. He showed me this last week and when I put our names together in the shape of a cross. Look it…matches…*(beaming).*

L/ Doctor: *(L sits in the chair N was sitting in)(interrupting)* Janet who showed you this?

N/JHC: Showed me? No one showed me anything Jesus is inside me.

L/ Doctor: Janet how long have you been feeling this way? Can you sit down for me? (slightly irritated)

N/JHC: I just feel so amazing. Like I could fly if I wanted.(*walking around and making movements with arms)* People are like little ants all walking around down there lost and not knowing that they are being controlled by the government…

L/ Doctor: Janet I am concerned that you have so much energy that you may hurt yourself. Have you been sleeping? What about eating?

N/JHC: I don't need to sleep as long as I can take my Lithium. Oh, yes please write me a prescription and I will be out of here. You look unhappy. The government has brain washed you….and…

LJ/ Doctor: *(interrupting and a little annoyed)* No Janet. No one has brain washed me… Please come and sit down. I would like to help you. Time-Out.*(N sit down in L's original seat and keeps writing disengaged from the scene.)*

Class?Comments? Using your interview template and checklist what information did I find out?

The audience/class responds with L in the role of the doctor and N (me) as the patient.

What is going on here beyond the fun that we have changing roles and locations? The content and format of the session apart from the role switching is very typical of a simulated patient teaching session in which a physician teacher role will model desired behaviour. Also the use of a template, the stopping and starting to ask questions and get observations from the student assemblage serves to engage their thinking and involvement. The switch which L and I enacted was one way of pointing up the fact that we are all performing in which ever role we take on in this encounter. Our identities are in fact fluid and multiple. We are performing different intersections of identities and the possibilities that accompany them. We are a desiring machine. Becoming –doctor–patient– standardized patient in a cartography that foregrounds our movement as "flows of matter" we are highlighting power issues endemic in ways of speaking and organizing thoughts attached to these different roles: The "doctor" asking questions and the "patient" responding (albeit with difficulty). In our action we are attempting to "deconstruct, and interrupt even momentarily the hubris of dominant cultural definitions of positions and roles as real and true" (Braidotti, 2009, p. 68).

The "difficult" in this encounter has to do with the doctor/interviewer's attempt to control the patient's pattern of information giving and its flow as a certain kind of story -a "clinical history" through questioning "techniques" which work only to a certain extent. On another level our improvised enactment of the physician role speaks to our familiarity as SPs with the doctor side of an interview and the sort of power that is implicitly shared in our SP role as complicit conmen. Teacher role modelling situations are always very difficult for SPs because we are aware that the physician may in fact not be modelling behaviour that as a real patient we might find helpful, and, in fact may find demeaning or disrespectful: yet we are located in such a way as to suggest an obligation to support the medical perspective through our performance and feedback. In this instance the audience/participants had "bought in" and were behaving as subjected medical trainees answering questions and responding as much as in any medical class in which I have been an SP.

7.3.2.1 Scene II

My colleague in her role as the doctor introduces the scenario of the depressed patient directing the class to the psychiatry interview hand-out andsets the stage to have one of the audience members come up to conduct part of the interview. I am seated quietly disengaged from the scene.

L/ Doctor: *(reading)* You are about to meet Elizabeth Scott. She has been brought into see you by her friend who is concerned that Elizabeth has missed work. She has told the nurse that when she visited Elizabeth at home she was shocked at the state of the apartment and at how haggard and very sad her friend looked. Elizabeth is a school teacher.

(to the audience) So. Who would like to come up and start the interview? This is the best seat in the house. You can time-out when ever you want and we will give you help. (*long silence*) We will up the ante. The first person up can choose a fellow classmate to come up after to continue the interview. (*Audience murmurs*). Remember you can't hurt the SP *(N. stands up and L hands her the lab coat, reflex hammerand stethoscope. *L. sits down in the patient chair and .N goes to the table and gets the stop watch and whistle).

N/Doctor *(picking up where L. left off)* *(cajoling)* They are not really experiencing anything *(pointing to the SP)* …. Better to try your hand here than with a real patient, remember you're being marked on participation.

This kind of patter about the "best seat in the house" in proximity to the mention of marks has manipulative edge to it. Unbelievably an audience member volunteers to begin the interview! Such role play exercises are described by students as nerve wracking as they attempt to take on the role of knowledgeable physician before their peers.

N/Doctor: Wonderful. I am going to time this as you will need to be aware of time for the organization of your interviewing, especially for your final examination – an OSCE. We can talk about that later. Before you start, what is your first question going to be? Class can we help her? *In fact I never use the watch but again it acts as a slightly threatening mechanism of control and power.*

C: *(A woman)* Um I don't know. I have never done this before. Ah....I guess I should find out more about her?

N/doctor: Exactly. Very good. We don't know if she is married or has children or how old she is. Is she on medications or been doing drugs? What else do we need to know? Class?

Silence – these are not the questions one asks at the start of a social encounter but rather fact finding questions. I am aware of feeling that this is very strange for all of us, myself included as the doctor, a role which is now starting to wear me down. I suggest a start. Why don't you ask her an open ended question like what has brought you in to the ER today? Or... tell me a little bit about yourself?

The interviewer does as I suggest. As the interview begins L. as the patient looks very sad, with downcast eyes and soft answers. The audience member student begins a conversation and then becomes lost and stops.

N/Doctor: Time-out. How was that for you?

C: I guess once I got started it was OK.

N/Doctor: Did you notice how your patient looks? Sounds?

C: Really sad. I was beginning to feel very badly for her.

N/doctor: Ah! Empathy.Excellent. We cover empathy next class. Thank you so much that was very brave and you made a wonderful start on getting to know your patient. Before we let you go back to your seat lets hear from our SP. *L. comes out of her patient role and introduces herself as the SP. She asks the woman how she felt she did and continues..*

L/SP: is there anything you would like to go back in and try again?

C: Ah No thank you.

L/SP: Do you have any questions for me? *(the woman shakes her head)* I appreciated your soft tone of voice when you spoke to me. It was very comforting. I also felt from your questions that you were really hearing what I was saying. So thank you.

N/doctor: (interrupting) We will have to work on tightening your organization or you won't get to all the important clinical information: but with practice. You did a very commendable first difficult interview. *(The woman sits down)* Who would like to go next? We have time for one more.

A woman puts up her hand and volunteers to come up. She later tells us that she is a nurse.

N/doctor: Thank you for volunteering. Where would you like to start?

D: I would like to find out if she is on any medications and if she has ever been seen for this before.

N/doctor: Great. I am going to time you. Time–in.

The audience member who is performing a medical student proceeds to do a wonderfully empathic interview in which she really does form a "therapeutic alliance" with L. as the patient. The interviewer timed out at one point to ask me a question that was a real clinical question about possible treatment options, for at this point she was not acting in any other capacity except as her nurse self. I felt disoriented as I moved from actor who was performing the role of a teaching doctor into small group teacher who was now trying to field questions as I might in any other similar teaching session as a SP facilitator. This meant that I redirected her clinical queries back to the process of the exchange. What was she hearing from the patient? What was her sense of the patient's safety? She had rightly brought up the question of suicide and of the patient wanting to kill herself. Often for trainees engaged in encounters with simulated depressed patients one of the most difficult things for a student to ask frankly about is the patient's desire to die which often gets avoided altogether or referred to euphemistically as a question of wanting to "hurt" oneself which is not the same thing.

As well there was L who had embodied at different times SP–patient– doctor, following the moves of the interviewer and me. I felt all of our vulnerability: the participant as a real life nurse performing a medical student, L. as the SP/actor/co workshop leader, and my own as the teacher/doctor. We were all engaged in a complex hybrid of multiplicity that was more about faith in each other and the process, than acting. We were not acting but rather responding from a particular location that was open to change at any time. "Bodies in time are embodied and embedded entities fully immersed in webs of complex interaction, negotiation, and transformation with and through other entities" (Braidotti, 2006, p. 154). Where the first interviewer had engaged as herself as an inexperienced medical student/audience member, this woman was engaged as herself as health professional and I was engaged in one of my roles as a facilitator and L. in one of hers as an SP. I felt the energy shifting into something very familiar and yet completely different. Afterwards speaking with L. she described a similar awareness and felt that at it this point there was a momentum that we could only follow and not intervene to change. The set SP protocol in teaching settings involves staying in role until invited to come out of the scenario in order to give feedback. It is easier for an interviewer to go back into an encounter if the patient hasn't switched identities to that of SP who is providing feedback from outside the role..

> *Becoming marks in fact a qualitative leap in the transformation of subjectivity and of its constitutive affects. It is a trip across different fields of perception, different spatio-temporal coordinates: mostly it transforms negativity into affirmative affects: pain into compassion, loss into a sense of bonding, isolation into care (*Braidotti, 2009, p.214).

7.3.2.2 Epilogue I

Still in the role of the teacher/doctor I invited my colleague to come out of her patient role. She introduced herself to the audience/interviewer as L (the SP but not yet as co workshop facilitator and actor of the various roles). We conducted feedback about the encounter the way we would in a SP teaching situation. First we asked the audience member/interviewer for her experience of the encounter, then L provided her perceptions as the SP followed by audience/classmates' observations and then my own as the facilitator (at the same time maintaining the persona of doctor/teacher). It was a difficult tension as we found ourselves in different levels of interaction. The audience member who had volunteered to play the medical student wanted specific feedback about how she performed in the interview (as a practicing nurse? Or a pretend medical student?), and we could feel the audience becoming confused with a qualitative shift in tone and vocabulary. We were all engaged in a rhizomatic endeavour in which as Braidotti suggests "the challenge is to destabilize dogmatic hegemonic exclusionary power structures at the very heart of the identity structures of the dominant subject through rhizomatic intervention" (Braidotti, 2006, p. 69). This was a mutational process for which there was no single end point. We engaged in a rhizomatic practice of setting out on a particular path (medical interviewing, doctor/ patient/SP/actor interactions), and through following different intensities created unique and immanent assemblages. Unexpected intersecting nodes (nurse, participant SP workshop facilitator) surfaced different generative tensions.

Our performance ended after I as the doctor still in role, thanked both the audience member and L for their good work and invited the audience/class to applaud both their classmates' (interviewer one and two) efforts. L.J and

I then took off our "costumes" and introduced ourselves. Except for L.J's introduction as the SP following the interviews and our patient names we had remained nameless throughout the entire workshop. As Nancy and L.J. we began a conversation with the group about their experience and thoughts.

7.3.3 Epilogue II: A dance not a march

The audience, we discovered were a mixture of performance artists, performance activists (my first medical student exchange), a philosophy professor, gender and cultural studies professor, a couple of social workers, the nurse, some other students, and an SP! The SP was an older woman who had just recently started working as an SP and I believe was largely confused by the whole thing.

None of our presentation was scripted and my recounting of what was said is not exact. My colleague and I had an outline for what we wanted to cover and the sequence of exercises. The specific phrases we used with respect to describing what SPs do and the ways of referring to the SP ("our SP") and the students came from years of experience hearing these exchanges in classes. Similar to the way we learn roles as SPs, for this we did not memorize lines or block movement ahead of time. My colleague and I and the participants all created an assemblage of: performers – audiences – observers – experts novices – women – men together in which as Deleuze and Guattari suggest, "every constellation of singularities and traits of expression deducted from the flow [are] selected, organized stratified – in such a way as to converge (consistency) artificially and naturally:...a veritable invention"(1986, 406). My colleague and I were "following" as were all of us in the room, the flow of affect and intention that was materializing as we went along.

So how are we to understand this matter-movement, this matter-energy, this matter flow, this matter in variation that enters assemblages and leaves them? (Deleuze and Guattari, 1986, 407)" This is performance as haecceity, as singular event in which affect as intensity creates inter-relationality on a model of mutual specification and collective becomings. We created a mutual space of learning within an imaginary over the course of the performance.

> The "imaginary" refers to a set of socially mediated practices which function as the anchoring point, albeit unstable and contingent, for identifications and therefore for identity formation. These practices act like interactive structures where desire as subjective yearning and agency in a broader socio-political sense are mutually shaped by one another (Braidotti, 2006, p. 86).

The performance activist in the audience who I early on treated as both a medical student and "difficult patient" spoke about the frustration and powerless she felt at not being able to take control of her role within the group structure and in relation to the performance. She described feeling both alienated and drawn to what she was participating in: probably not unlike the experience of many medical students. It was a moment of rupture in which the "real" rubbed up against the representational, disrupting her role as a spectator and producing the possibility of new meanings. Observations can induce powerful discomfort that work as a challenges to assumed reality. "Participation in performances in which one is subjected is also powerful re-inscriptions of embodied truths" (Reinhart, 2010, p. 173).

The philosophy professor who entered the space late spoke about the palpable power differential he felt as he walked into the room even before I addressed him. This did not feel to him like a regular audience watching a performance. He felt pre - subjected as a certain kind of audience participant: the entitled medical student before he said or did anything. The numerous handouts were also confounding for him as he tried to figure out what he was expected to know. A demand for presence as outlined in the first page of the syllabus, with no information about the behaviour being referred to —*"Behaviour inconsistent with being a physician is viewed as a demonstration of lack of suitability to be a physician"* – is also part of a cultural apparatus of medical education as a hierarchical machine.

Some of the discussion we engaged in as a group at the end covered issues about the "not real" nature of the work in which SPs engage, their status as "not really" experiencing entities, the complicit constitutive role that SPs take on with respect to medical education and professional identity formation. There was affirmation from the group that the critical space we all created brought to life a rich embodied material performance of contingent identity formations. "Unmasking realness for representation and visa versa does not undo the power but rather compels a different model of understanding about the relation of the real to representation" (Reinelt, 2010, p. 174). Such an understanding about the contingent nature of our professional roles and day to day lives acknowledges that ambiguity is not a problem but a starting place.

7.4 Performance

As a political undertaking such performances hinge on ideas about identity, subjectivity, agency and power as sites of contestation and play. According to a Deleuzian ontology of becoming we find ourselves on a plane of immanence.

> Perception will no longer reside in the relation between the subject and an object, but rather in the movement serving as a limit of that relation…. Perception will confront its own limit; it will be in the midst of things, throughout its own proximity, as the presence of one haecceity in another,… Look only at the movements (Deleuze & Guattari, 1987, p. 282).

Performance as a form of ethics then is always taking place in the movement between positions, locations, and subjectivities, facilitating cross border connections and alliances among "differentially located constituencies which in itself becomes a political position" (Braidotti, 2006, p.67). As described by Braidotti the point of such activity is not just mere deconstruction but the relocation of identities on new grounds that account for multiple belongings, i.e. a non unitary vision of the subject (p. 69). This is a collective and affective undertaking which "as a project requires active participation and enjoyment; a new virtual love which targets less what we are, more what we are capable of becoming" (p.87).

7.4.1 Performance as Nomadic ethics

"Nomadism as a counter-method starts from the politics of location. This is both a strategy and a method based on politically charged cartographies of one's position, starting not from gender alone but from a bundle of interrelated social relations" (Braidotti, 2009, p. 92). As nomads, SPs perform not only patient roles but also various "locations" within a medical education system. We are not merely acting as generic containers into which values and ideas can be poured. As "perpetually possible" educational partners we retain situated perspectives in terms of gender, sexual identity, race, class age and other historically informed coordinates. "Nomadic subjects are not quantitative pluralities but rather qualitative multiplicities" (Braidotti, 2006, p. 58). As such SPs express changes not of scale but of intensity, force or potential.

This location of multiple intensive variables allows movement between unknown territories of becoming. "The politics of location like nomadism is both material and immanent. As a method it combines issues of self reflexivity and accountability with ways of enlarging scientific objectivity. "It involves dialogical confrontations with others in a mixture of affectivity/involvement and objectivity/distance which needs to be balanced in a critical manner" (Braidotti, 2006, p. 93).

7.4.2 Emotion and Affect as Aesthetic Performance

> Vulnerability becomes strength only when the performer can fracture all the technique that has been built up - to allow the shadow to emerge – abandon it – exposing herself like a warrior who fights with bare hands (Barba, 1995, p. 65).

Performance always entails a reach across a gap or the negotiation of a crack that is permanent as an absent presence. Such a pause or break holds a potential affective charge. It "is a movement of intention that is immobile, silent: the cat that is doing nothing yet, but we understand is about to pounce. It is a felt charge and a moment of transition that leads to a new precise posture" (Barba, 1995, p. 56). As such performing is not a question of representativeness or validity but of connecting relationally with a continually shifting unknown. It is a giving up of the technical and epistemological knowns in order to take the risk of exposing oneself anew in each situation. As opposed to a narcissistic exercise of self transformation in the interests of attaining more or different visibility for its own sake, the process which my colleague and I undertook through performance was crucially about imagination and interconnection. "Learning to undo things and to undo oneself, is proper to the war machine: the "not doing" of the warrior, the undoing of the subject" (Deleuze & Guattari, 1986, p. 400). Such a process is a form of transformation premised on the possibility of becoming that is open ended. Creating a space in which not knowing and failure was possible was crucial, to our undertaking but so also was creating opportunities for play.

The ontology put forward by Deleuze and Guattari is essentially affirmatively creative and committed to the productive power of desire and joy. These are not the empty prescriptions of a simplistic E.I. model in which joy is the method by which one attains greater success or wealth. For performers a creative space of productive potential engages energy as positive force. Barba suggests: "Above and beyond the metaphorical uses to which it can be put, the word energy implies a difference of potential. Geographers for example, refer to the energy of a region to indicate the arithmetic difference between maximum and minimum heights. He continues: "The Greek word enérghia means to be ready for action" (Barba, 1995, p.55). This evokes the felt sense of affective power as immanent and the possibility of creativity in indeterminate spaces.

Performance as an ethical and aesthetic process of learning is a form of metamorphosis or mutation. It is evocative in the richest sense of the word. Just as for Deleuze and Guattari "becoming imperceptible" involves a pragmatic ethics and an invitation to stretch to the limit of his or her capacity" (1986, p. 202), for the actor, crossing borders and living in the moment and on the margins in perpetual liminality is a nomadic path of interconnection. Movement as intensity alone is an affective undertaking. Learning envisioned as a process of becoming is likewise a liminal experience that involves mourning the loss of certainty and as such is an affective and emotional undertaking. In all of these endeavours the invisible yet present force of desire is an energy that we imbue with the most poignant hopes. "Energy is a personal temperature – intensity which the performer can determine, awaken, model" (Barba, 1995, p. 62). The affective power of acting/performing is a process of flows of becoming and of heightened perception and receptivity. In describing the process of becoming a performer, Barba uses terminology reminiscent of Deleuze and Guattari's description of becoming a nomad war machine:

> They are working on something invisible: energy. The experienced performer learns not to associate energy mechanically with an excess of muscular or nervous energy, but with something intimate something which pulsates with immobility and silence, and a retained power-thought which grows in time without manifesting itself in space (Barba, 1995, p. 56).

7.4.3 SP Performances and Transpositions

I have described a different kind of performance and one which is unique with respect to the kind of work in which SPs usually engage. The project was an attempt to create a particular assemblage of embodied media within which to explore effects of power as they play out from different perspectives. It was a risky undertaking which involved vulnerability which I feel even in reconstructing it here. There were many possibilities for some of the many border crossings to have sparked resentment or anger. As described by Braidotti we attempted a "transposition": a leap from one coda, field, or axis to another. She states

> As a term in music, transposition indicates variations and shifts of scale in a discontinuous but harmonious pattern. It is thus created as an in-between space of zigzagging and of crossing: non linear, but not chaotic, nomadic, yet accountable and committed; creative but also cognitively valid; discursive and also materially embedded – it is coherent without falling into instrumental rationality (Braidotti, 2006, p. 5).

This describes for me the intent of our overall project and acknowledges our role changing as well as our different interactions with each other and with the audience/participants. For me an intimacy and care for the "students'" experiences is a different quality of relationship than one of performer to audience and different yet again from teacher to student. Empathy and the effects of its lack in the space which we created was also tangible. I felt the group's varying engagement, confusion, frustration and fellow feeling, like vibrating cord running between us. My fellow actor and friend and I were "both/and" in our relational exchanges; as we are in our day to day life; multiple selves not acting *per se* but performing choices as accountable across multiple lines of becoming.

Deleuze and Guattari might identify our assemblage as constituting a kind of "machinic phylum", referring to a particular constellation of singularities with its own operations, qualities and traits. "Such constellations determine the relation of desire to the technical element (the affects the sabre "has" are not the same as those of the sword)" (Deleuze & Guattari, 1987, p. 406). So, just as the sabre and the sword are ostensibly the same kind of weapon with apparently the same qualities and functions, their genealogy, materials and relationships as weapons are affectively and qualitatively different. Much like actors and SPs who, although ostensibly genetically of the same family with roots in performance, have over time qualitatively and affectively become aligned slightly differently to their work.

> In the time between the doing and the thing done, however give or take 'the blink of an eye' performance theorists see 'what Plato condemned in theatrical representation' – its non originality – and gesture toward an epistemology grounded not on the distinction between truthful models and fictional representations but on different ways of knowing and doing that are constitutively heterogeneous,

contingent and risky (E. Diamond 1996, cited in Roach, 2010, p. 457).

7.5 Conclusion

Will such performances as educational events be valuable or possible in other educational settings? Although SP teaching sessions always involve improvisation and moment by moment following as in the performance just described, the different levels at which the role play took place in this instance was unique in my experience. I am never pretending to be a doctor teaching a group of pretend medical students in my work as an SP teacher. The New York cityworkshop experience was a bit like playing with fire in that we didn't know until we were engaged in its unfolding what mutual lessons might emerge or get lost or misunderstood. But don't we struggle with the same concerns in learning situations in which affect apparently has no place? Engaged pedagogy is always on the threshold between the known and unknown. What I discovered over the course of both creating and performing this event together with my colleague was an approach to bringing theory to life literally, into an affective space and making implicit power relations explicit through the lived medium of performance. Opportunities for immediate critical exploration of the participants' experiences of different ideas not simply their thinking about them, added a dimension to our learning that included an ethics of effects. Each of us brings our entire lives into learning situations not just our brains and we make decisions about which roles we believe are necessary and right based on multiple factors. How these decisions play out and their effects on others is central to our day to day lives and the affirmative role we as educators can play in making visible inequities that hide in theoretical models developed to privilege the few. This affective embodiment of theory through play was also an engagement of human simulation as creative subversion. As a living methodology with the power to reveal and embody the effects of ideas such practices hold much educational promise.

Notes

1. My sincere gratitude to my dear friend and colleague Laura Jayne Nelles for our many rich conversations about our work as SPs and for the creative time we spent engaged in this performance piece. I am most indebted to her for her permission to share it as part of my thesis.

PROCESS CHECKLIST	

Fill in the box which best reflects your judgement of the student's performance in the following categories

Student's response to patient's feelings and needs (empathy).

☐　　☐　　☐　　　　☐　　☐

Does **not** responds to obvious patient cues *and/or* responds **inappropriately.**	Responds to patient's cues, but not always effectively.	Responds **consistently** in a **perceptive,** and **genuine** manner to the patient's needs and cues.

Degree of coherence in the interview.

☐　　☐　　☐　　　☐　　☐

No recognizable plan to the interaction, the plan does **not** demonstrate cohesion, *or* the **patient** must determine the direction of the interview.	Organizational approach is **formulaic and minimally flexible** *and/or* control of the interview is **inconsistent.**	**Superior organization,** demonstrating **command** of cohesive devises, **flexibility,** and **consistent control** of the interview.

Verbal Expression

☐ ☐ ☐ ☐ ☐

Communicates in manner that **interferes with** *and/or***prevents understanding** by patient	Exhibits **suffcient control** of expression to be **understood** by an active listener (patient)	Exhibits **command** of expression (fluency, grammar, vocabulary, tone, volume and modulation of voice, rate of speech, pronunciation.

Non-Verbal Expression

☐ ☐ ☐ ☐ ☐

Fails to engage, frustrates*and/or* antagonizes the patient.	Exhibits **enough control** of non-verbal expression to **engage** a patient willing to overlook deficiencies such as passivity, self-consciousness, or inappropriate aggressiveness.	Exhibits **finesse and command** of non-verbal expression (eye contact, gesture, posture, use of silence).

Based on your clinical impression, did this student demonstrate competence at the level of a clerk in this situation? Do not add up the check marks. Rather, base it on your GLOBAL impression of the performance

NOT COMPETENT ☐	BORDERLINE ☐	COMPETENT ☐
Student Name:		

Examiner Comments:

2. The handouts are actual documents used in teaching communication skills and are the property of the University of Toronto Standardized Patient Program, available on the web site www.spp.utoronto.ca.

Chapter 8 Final Reflections

"We are all just slipping glimpsers" (deKooning)

8.0 Reflections

This has been a very different undertaking from the one I set out on. The alternative path that I have followed through the story of SPs as informed by Deleuze and Guattari, Foucault, and the thinking of feminist poststructuralist perspectives about emotion and affect, leaves me feeling like I am standing in new territory. How might such an alternative reading contribute to the field of medical education, the field of human simulation and education more broadly from this location?

The location of SPs within medical education is both a place of great freedom and limitation, and one which is continually changing as new technologies emerge and new relationships are imagined for applications of experiential learning. Exploration of the ethical and practical implications of these various relationships is largely uncharted territory in health professional education as they are, I would suggest, in the area performance arts and even the larger field of education. The work of SPs and the teaching we undertake is about possibility, activated through inhabiting different stories and by connecting them affectively to larger social concerns. I have come to appreciate more fully the crucial role that a practical ethics of emotion and affect play in the embodied work of SPs. But more importantly my exploration has made visible for me how emotion and affect as political forces are implicated with respect to SPs complex desire for legitimacy within a profession that shapes the field in which they work and subjects them as valued helpmates.

Education is an ethical undertaking and as such requires conversations and multiple perspectives. It is a project of political praxis that recognizes the effects of knowledge production as materially implicated – on real bodies and lives. Such a recognition calls for us to recognize the educational consequences of generosity and compassion in our approach as teachers. Paying attention to and ensuring that the relationships and dialogues that we make possible in simulation learning situations are real even if the bodies increasingly may not be, I see as important undertaking. In this way performance as an aesthetic activity creates opportunities to introduce and mull over issues related to affect and emotion as central forces of learning.

Enacting education along nomadic paths means acknowledging that exteriorized and excluded elements such as desire and passion are forces that make all of our endeavours messy, more real and richer than when we attempt to lock them in place. It is in the "in between" of our educational pursuits and not at their end points or beginnings that we stand as teachers to make the most difference. The many instances where we fail and make attempts that don't materialize our expectations of perfection are fertile sites of learning: Although these are not comfortable or easy.

Like crabgrass that proliferates rhizomatically, connecting generatively to new life forms, different educational opportunities are attended by unintended and unseen consequences. My appreciation for education as a site of perpetual imperfection and creative possibilities directs me towards introducing practices that recognize the creative potency of learning and the possibilities that can emerge unexpectedly from real places of mutual struggle and celebration. As Jamie Magnusson suggests, "a nomadic practice in education requires working toward mutually nourishing relationships in the process of dismantling relationships that hierarchize and subjectify" (Magnusson, 2011, p. 158).

We don't know the possibilities that different ideas about emotion and affect might proliferate, or how integrating knowledges from a range of epistemological traditions and ontological perspectives might change our practices as educators.

Education is an embodied cultural and political undertaking that shapes and is shaped by emotion and affect. Within health professional education, rethinking emotion and affect as epistemological and philosophical concerns has the possibility of inspiring new research that challenges taken for granted notions of professionalism and professional socialization processes, while at the same time contributing to a growing field of inquiry. Within the larger field of education I look forward to joining conversations that include questions about embodied and embedded ethics as both practice and method of theoretical concern.

References

Abrahamson, S., Denson, J.S., Wolf, R.M. (1969). Effectiveness of a simulator in training anaesthesiology residents.*Journal of Medical Education,* 44, 515-519.

Ahmed, S. (2004). *The cultural politics of emotion.* New York: Routledge.

Albuquerque, J. (June 26, 2007) When doctors cry.*The Globe and Mail,* Toronto, Ontario: Philip Crowley Publisher, L5.

Anderson, M.B., Kassenbaum, D.G. (Eds.). (1993). Special Issue: Proceedings of the AAMC's Consensus Conference on the Use of Standardized Patients in the Teaching and Evaluation of Clinical Skills. *Academic Medicine,* 68, 437-483.

Aristotle, *Aristotle's Poetics.* (1961). (S.H. Butcher,Trans.) New York: Hill and Wang.

Ashkanazy, N.M., Daus, C. (2005). Rumors in the death of emotional intelligence in organizational behavior are vastly exaggerated. *Journal of Organizational Behavior,* 26, 441-452.

Barba, E. (1995). *The paper canoe: A Guide to theatre Anthropology.* (Richard Fowler, Trans.). London, New York: Routledge.

Bar-On, R. (1997). B*ar-On Emotional Quotient Inventory (EQI). Technical Manual,* Toronto: Multi Health Systems.

Barrows, H. S., Abrahamson, S. (1964). The programmed patient: A technique for Appraising Student Performance in Clinical Neurology. *Journal of Medical Education,* 39, 802-805.

Barrows, H.S. (1968). Simulated patients in medical training.*Canadian Medical Association Journal*, IV(98), 674-676.

Barrows, H.S. (1971). *Simulated patients (programmed patients): development and use of a new technique in medical education*. Springfield Il: Thomas.

Barrows, H.S. (1987). *Simulated (Standardized Patients) and other human simulations.*Chapel Hill: Health Sciences Consortium.

Barrows, H. (1993). An overview of the uses of standardized patients for teaching and Evaluating Clinical Skills.*Academic Medicine,* 68(6), 443-451.

Barrow, H. (1999). *Training standardized patients to have physical findings.* (self published hand book, 32 pages).

Baudrillard, J. (1983). *Simulations*.(P. Foss, P. Patton, and P. Beitchman, Trans.). New York: Semiotext[e].

Becker, H.S. (2004). *Boys in white: Student culture in medical School.* (eighth ed.). New Brunswick (USA) and London (U.K.):Transaction Publishers.

Belling, C. (2009).Endography: A physician's dream of omniscience. In E. Klaver (Ed.), *The Body on Medical Culture.* p. 151-173. New York: SUNY Press.

Best, S., Kellner, D. (1991). *Postmodern theory: Critical interrogations.* New York: The Guildford Press.

Bhaba, H. (1987). Interrogating identity. In: L. Appignaesi (Ed.), *Identity.*p.5-11. London: Institute of Contemporary Art.

Bleakley, A., Bligh, J., Browne, J. (2011). *Medical education for the future: Identity, power and location.* Dordrecht. Heidelberg. London. New York: Springer.

Bleakley, A. (2006). Broadening conceptions of learning in medical education: the message from teamworking.*Medical Education,* 40, 150-157.

Bligh, J., Bleakley, A. (2006). Distributing menus to hungry learners: can learning by simulation become simulation of learning. *Medical Teacher.*28(7), 606-613.

Boal, A. (1979) invisible theatre.*Adult Education and Development.* 12, 29-31.

Boler, M. (December, 1996). *Assembled emotions and mutant affects: Towards a semiotics of (un) domesticated feeling.* p. 1-27. Presented at Deleuze: A Symposium,.University of Western Australia, Perth.

Boler, M. (1997).Disciplined emotions: Philosophies of educated feelings.*Education. Theory*, 4; 203-227.

Boler, M. (1999).*Feeling power: Emotions and education*. New York. London: Routledge.

Bligh. J., Parsell. G. (1999). Research in medical education: Finding its place. *Medical Education,* 33(3), 162–163.

Bradley, P. (2006). The history of simulation in medical education and possible future directions.*Medical Education,* 40, 254-262.

Braidotti, R. (1996/2011).*Nomadic subjects: gender and culture.* (2nd edition). New York: Columbia University Press.

Braidotti, R. (2006). *Transpositions: On nomadic ethics.* Cambridge, U.K: Polity.

Bruer, J.T. (1997). Education and the brain: A bridge too far, *Educational Researcher,* 4-16.

Brosnan, C., Turner, B. (2009). *Handbook of the sociology of medical education.*London and New York: Routledge Taylor and Francis Group.

Bryden, P., Ginsburg S., Kurabi, B., Ahmed, N. (2010). Professing professionalism: Are we our own worst enemy? Faculty members' experiences of teaching and evaluating professionalism in medial education in one school.*Academic Medicine*, 85: 1-10.

Buck, G.H. (1991). Development of simulators in medical education.*Gesnerus,* 48(1), 7 – 28.

Buckman, R. (2002). Communications and emotions: Skills and effort are key. *British Medical Journal,* 325: 672-4.

Butler, J. (2005). *Giving an account of oneself.* New York: Fordham University Press.

Canadian Theatre Encyclopaedia. Retrieved May, 10, 2011, from .http://www.canadiantheatre.com/dict.pl?term=Waiting%20for%20the%20Parade.

Carrothers, R.M., Gregory, S.W., Gallagher, T.J. (2000). Measuring emotional intelligence of medical school applicants. *Academic Medicine,* 75: 456-61.

Cassells, J. (1996). The woman in the surgeon's body.*American Anthropologist,* 98 (1), 41-53.

Cherryholmes, C.H. (1988). *Power and criticism: Post structural investigations in education.* New York, London: Teachers College Press.

Clarke, N. (1993). From playthings to professionals: The English actress from 1660-1990. *Gender and History,* 15(1), 120-124.

Clough, P.T. (2007). *The affective turn.*Durham and London: Duke University Press.

Cohen, S. (1983).The Mental hygiene movement, The development of personality and the school: The medicalization of American education. *History of Education Quarterly,* 23(2) 123-149.

Colebrook, C. (2006). *Deleuze: A guide for the perplexed.* London, New York, Continuum Press.

Colliver, J., Conlee, M., Verhulst, S., Dorsey, K. (2010). Reports on the decline of empathy during medical education are greatly exaggerated: A re-examination of the research. *Academic Medicine,* 85, (4), 588-593.

Conquergood, D. (1995). Of caravans and carnivals: Performance studies in motion. *TDR: The Drama Review*, 39 (4), 137-141.

Cooper, J.B., Taqueti, V.R. (2004). A brief history of the mannequin simulators for clinical education and training.*Quality and Safety in Health Care,* 13, 11-18.

Coulehan, J. (2006). You say self interest, I say altruism, in *Professionalism in Medicine: Critical Perspectives*. (Eds) D. Wear and J. Aultman. p. 103-127. New York:Springer.

Damasio, A. R. (1994). *Descartes error: emotion, reason, and the human brain.* New York: Avon Books.

Daniels, M. (1960).Affect and its control in the medical intern.*American Journal of Sociology,* 55:259-67.

Darwin, C. (1872). *The expression of the emotions in man and animals.*London: Murray.

Davis, T. (1991).*Actresses as working women: Their social identity in victorian culture.* Oxford, New York: Routledge.

Deleuze, G. (1970/1988).*Spinoza: practical philosophy.* (R. Hurley, Trans.). San Francisco: City Light Books.

Deleuze, G. (1989). *Cinema 2: The time image.* (H. Tomlinson & R. Galeta, Trans.) Minneapolis: University of Minnesota Press.

Deleuze, G., Parnet, C. (1987). *Dialogues*. (H. Tomlinson & B. Habberjam, Trans.). London: Athlone. p.74.

Deleuze, G., Guattari, F. (1987/2005). *A thousand plateaus: capitalism and schizophrenia.* (B. Massumi, Trans.). Minneapolis & London: University of Minnesota Press.

DeMaria, S., Bryson, E.O., Mooney, T.J., Silverstein, J.H., Reich, D.L., Bodian, C., Levine, A.I. (2010). Adding emotional stressors to training in simulated cardiopulmonary arrest enhances participant performance. *Medical Education,* 44(1), 1006-1015.

Department of Health. (2000). *An organisation with a memory.* London: Stationery Office.

Descartes, R. (1649/1989).*Passions of the soul.*(S. Voss, Trans. and annotated). Indianapolis: Hackett Publishing.

Diamond, E. (Ed.) (1996).*Performance and cultural politics.* New York. Routledge.

Diderot, D. (1970). Le paradoxesur le comedien.In T. Cole, & H.K. Chinoy, (Eds.).*Actors on Acting: The theories, techniques and practices of the world's great actors*162-170.New York: Three Rivers Press.

Didi-Hubeman, G. (1982/2003).*Invention of hysteria: Charcot and the photographic iconography of the Salpêtrière.* (A. Hartz, Trans.). Cambridge, MA, London, U.K: MIT Press.

Diedrich, L. (2007). *Treatments: Language, politics and the culture of illness.* Minneapolis & London: University of Minnesota Press.

Dixon, T. (2003).*From passions to emotions: The creation of a secular psychological category.* Cambridge U.K.: Cambridge University Press.

Dormans, J. (2008). *Beyond iconic simulation.*http://www.jorisdormans.nl/article.php?ref=beyondiconicsimulation. Retrieved April 7 2011.

Dreyfus, H., Rabinow, P. (1982/1983).*Michel Foucault: Beyond structuralism and hermeneutics* (second ed.). Chicago: University of Chicago Press.

Elam, C., Stratton, T.D., Andrykowski, M.A. (2001). Measuring the emotional intelligence of medical school matriculents.*Academic Medicine,* 76: 507-508.

Ellaway, R., Poulton, T., Fors, U., McGee, J., Albright, S. (2008). Building a virtual patient commons. *Medical Teacher*; 30(2),170-74.

Elllsworth, E. (1989). Why Doesn't this feel empowering. In *Feminisms and Critical Pedagogy,* New York, NY, London, UK: Routledge.

Feldman, M.D. (2001). Becoming an emotionally intelligent physician.*Western Journal of Medicine*, 175(2): 98.

Filkins, D., Burns, J.F. (2006). The reach of war: Military deep in a U.S. dessert, practicing to face the Iraq insurgency. *New York Times,* 1May. http://query.nytimes.com/gst/fullpage.html?res=9D0DE6DD113FF932A35 76C0A9609C8B63&n=Top/Reference/Times%20Topics/People/F/Filkins, %20Dexter. Retrieved 21 Nov, 2010.

Fletcher, G.C.L., McGeorge, P., Flin, R.H., Glavin, R.J., Maran N.J. (2002). The role of non technical skills in anaesthesia: A Review of the current literature. *British Journal of Anaesthesia,* 88(3) 418 – 429.

Flexner, A. (1910). *Medical education in the United States and Canada: A report to the Carnegie foundation for the advancement of teaching.* Boston, MA: Updyke.

Foucault, M. (1969).*The archaeology of knowledge and the discourse on language*. (A.M. Sheridan, Trans.). London, UK. Routledge Classics.

Foucault, M. (1972/1980).*Power/Knowledge selected interviews and other writings* 1972-1977.New York, Random House.

Foucault, M. (1976). Two lectures. In C Gordon, (ed.) *Power/Knowledge: Selected Interviews and other Writings*, p. New York. Pantheon Books Ltd.

Foucault, M. (1977).*Language, counter memory, practice.*New York. Cornell University Press.

Foucault, M. (1977/1995).*Discipline & punish: The birth of the prison*. (A. M. Sheridan Trans.). New York: Vintage Books.

Foucault, M. (1977/1980).*language, counter-memory, practice: selected essays and interviews.*D. Bouchard, (Ed.). Ithica, NY: Cornell Press.

Foucault, M. (1978/1980).*The History of sexuality, Volume 1: an introduction.*(R. Hurley, Trans.).New York: Random House.

Foucault, M. (1981)."The Order of Discourse," In Young R, (Ed.) *Untying the text: A poststructuralist reader*. London, UK: Routledge and Kegan Paul.

Foucault, M. (1982). Afterword: The subject and power in *Michel Foucault: Beyond structuralism and hermeneutics* (second ed.) p. 208-226. Chicago, IL: University of Chicago Press.

Foucault, M. (1984).*The Foucault Reader,* P. Rabinow, (ed.). London, UK, New York, NY: Penguin.

Foucault, M. (1996).*Foucault Live: Interviews 1961-1984.* S. Lotringer,. (Ed.). New York, NY: Semotext(e).

Foucault, M. (1997/2003).*Society must be defended: Lectures at the College de France 1975-1976.* A. Davidson, (English Series Ed.). (D. Macey, Trans.). New York, NY: Picador.

Frank, J. (1996). Skills for the new iillennium: Report of the societal needs working group, CanMEDS 2000 Project. *Annals Royal College of Physicians and Surgeons of Canada, 29,* 206-216.

Frank, J. Danoff, D. (2007). The CanMEDS initiative: Implementing an outcomes based framework of physician competencies. *Medical Teacher,* 29, 642-647.

Friedman, Z.,You-Ten, K.E., Bould, M.D., Naik, V. (2008). Teaching lifesaving procedures: the impact of model fidelity on acquisition and transfer of cricothyrotomy skills to performance on cadavers. *Anaesthesia Analgesia.* 107(5),1663-9.

Gardner, H.(1985). *The mind's new science.* New York: Basic Books.

Gilman, S.(1993). The image of the hysteric, In *Hysteria beyond Freud* 345-452. Berkeley, LA, London, UK: University of California Press.

Godkins, T. (1974).Utilization of simulated patients to teach routine pelvic examination.*AcademicMedicine.*49(12),1174-8.

Goffan, E. (1961).The self and social roles. In *Encounters: Two Studies in the Sociology of Interaction,* Indianapolis, IN: Bobbs-Merill.

Good, B. J. (2003). *Medicine, rationality and experience: An anthropological perspective*. New York: Cambridge University Press.

Good, D., Byron-Good, M.J. (1993). Learning medicine: The constructing of medical knowledge at Harvard Medical School.In*Knowledge, Power and Practice*. S. Lindbaum, & M. Lock, (Eds.). Berkeley, CA: University of California Press.

Gordon, RB. (2004). From Charcot to Charlot: Unconscious imitation and spectatorship in French cabaret and early cinema. In: M. Micale (Ed.), *The mind of modernism* 93 – 125. Stanford, CA. Stanford Press.

Gould, S.J, (1981/1996). *The mismeasure of man*. New York, NY, London, UK: W.W. Norton & Company.

Goleman, D. (1995). *Emotional Intelligence*.New York.Bantam Books.

Greene, M, (1973). *Teacher as stranger*.Belmont CA. Wadsworth Publishing Company Inc.

Grosz, E. (1994). *Volatile bodies: Toward a corporeal feminism.* Indianapolis & Bloomington, IN: Indiana University Press.

Grosz, E. (1993). Bodies and knowledges: Feminism and the crisis of reason. In.L. Alcoff& E. Potter (Eds), *Feminism and the crisis of reason infeminist epistemologies* 187-217. New York: Routledge.

Hafferty, F. (2000). In search of a lost cord: Professionalism and medical education's hidden curriculum. In D. Wear and J. Bickel (Eds.), *Educating for Professionalism: Creating a culture of humanism in medical education* 11-34. Iowa City, Iowa: University of Iowa Press.

Hafferty, F, Castellani, B. (2009). The Hidden Curriculum: A theory of medical education. In C. Brosnan& B. Turner (Eds.), *Handbook of the sociology of medical education* 9 – 35. London, UK, New York, NY: Routledge Taylor and Francis Group.

Hall, S. (1997). *Representation: Cultural representations and signifying practices.* London, UK: Sage Publications.

Hanna, M., Fins, J, (2006). Power and communication: Why simulation training ought to be complemented by experiential and humanist learning. *Academic Medicine*, 81(3), 265-270.

Haraway, D. (1991). A cyborg manifesto: Science, technology, and socialist-feminism in the late twentieth century. In *Simians, cyborgs and women: The reinvention of nature* 149-181. New York, NY: Routledge.

Harden, R.M., Gleeson, F.A. (1979). Assessment of clinical competence using an observed structured clinical examination.*Medical Education,* 13, 41-47.

Hardt, M. (2007). Foreword: What are affects good for? In P T. Clough, J. Halley (Eds.), *The affective turn* (p.ix- xiii). Durham & London, UK: Duke University Press.

Harris, S.B. (1992).The society for the recovery of persons apparently dead.*Skeptic.*1, 24-31.

Hayles, K. (1993). Virtual bodies and flickering signifiers.*OCTOBER,* 66, 61-69.

Hillman, J. (1960). *Emotion: A comprehensive phenomenology of theories and their meanings for therapy*. Evanston, Ill: North Western University Press.

The Hippocratic Oath".National Institute of Health.Retrieved April 5, 2010. http://www.nlm.nih.gov/hmd/greek/greek_oath.html.

Hochschild, A,R. (2003). *The managed heart: commercialization of human feeling* (11th ed.).Berkeley, CA: University of California Press.

Hodges, B. (2003). OSCE variations on a theme by Harden.*Medical Education*, 37(12), 1134-1140.

Hodges, B. (2004). Medical student bodies and the pedagogy of self reflection, self assessment and self regulation.*Journal of Curriculum Theorizing,* 20(2), 41-51.

Hodges, B., (2005). The many and conflicting histories of medical education in Canada and the United States: An introduction to the paradigm wars. *Medical Education, 39(*6).613-621.

Hodges, B., (2006). Medical education and the maintenance of Incompetence.*Medical Teacher,* 28, 690-696.

Hodges, B., (2009). *The Objective Structured Clinical Examination: A Socio-History*. Köln, Germany: LAP LAMBERT Academic Publishing AG & Co. KG..

Hojat, M., Mangione, S., Nasca, T.J. (2004).An empirical study of the decline in empathy in medical school.*Medical Education,* 38, 934-941.

hooks, b. (1994). *Teaching to transgress.*New York, London: Routledge.

Human Patient Simulation Network websitehttp://www.hpsn.com/event/hpsn-annual-2012/67/#tab_workshopsandcourses.Retrieved July 12, 2011.

Issenberg, S.B., McGaghie, W.C., Petrusa, E.R., Lee, G. D., Scalese, R.J. (2005).Features and uses of high-fidelity medical simulations that lead to effective learning: a BEME systematic review. *Medical Teacher*; 27(1), 10-28.

Jaggar, A. (1989). Love and knowledge: Emotion in feminist epistemology. *Inquiry*, 32, 151-176.

Joughin, M. (1990).*Negotiations:Gilles Deleuze*. New York, NY: Columbia University Press.

Kao, A., Reenan, J. (2006). *WIT* is not enough. In *Professionalism in Medicine: critical perspectives* 211-232. D. Wear and J. Aultman(Eds.),New York, NY: Springer.

Katritzky, M.A. (2007). *Women, medicine and theatre 1500-1750: Literary mountbanks and performing quacks.* Aldershot, U.K: Ashgate Publishing.

Keenoy, T., Oswick, C., Grant, D., (1997). Organizational discourses: Text and context, *Organization, 2*, 147-158.

Kemper, T.D., (1993). Sociological models in the explanation of emotions. In: *Handbook of Emotions* 41-51. M. Lewis, J.M. Haviland (Eds.). New York, NY: The Guilford Press.

Kendall, G., Wickham, G. (2003). *Using Foucault's method*. London: Sage Publications.

King, H. (1993). Once Upon a Text: Hysteria from Hippocrates. In *Hysteria beyond Freud* 3 -91. S. Gilman (Ed.), Berkeley, CA, Los Angeles, CA, London, UK: University of California Press.

Klamen, D., Williams, R. (2006). Using standardized clinical encounters to assess physician communication. In D. T. Stern (Ed.), *Measuring Professionalism* (p. 53-75). Oxford, UK New York, NY: Oxford University Press.

Kneebone, R., Nestel, D., Yadollahi, F., Brown, R., Nolan, C., Durack, J., Brenton, H., Moulton, C., Archer, J., &Darzi, A. (2006). Assessing procedural skills in context: Exploring the feasibility of an Integrated Procedural Performance Instrument (IPPI). *Medical Education*; 40, 1105-1114.

Kohn, L.T., Corrigan, J.M., Donaldson, M.S. (2000). *To err Is human: Building a safer health system*. Washington, DC: National Academy Press.

Lather, P. (1991).*Getting smart: feminist research and pedagogy with/in the post modern*. New York, NY. London, UK: Routledge.

Lazarus, R.S. (1991). *Emotion and adaptation.* New York, NY: Oxford University Press.

LeBlanc,V.R., Tavares, W., King,K., Scott,A.K., Macdonald,R., Regehr, C. (2010). The impact of stress on paramedic performance during simulated critical events.*Simulation in Healthcare,* 5(6), 440.

LeDoux, J., (1996). *The Emotional brain: The mysterious underpinnings of emotional Life.* New York, NY: Simon & Schuster.

Lewis, B. (2006). Medical professionalism and the discourse of professionalism: Teaching complications. In D. Wear and J. Aultman (Eds.), *Professionalism in medicine: Critical perspectives* 149-165. New York, NY: Springer.

Lieff, H.I., Fox, R.C. (1963). Training for "detached concern" in medical students. In H.I. Lieff, V.F. Lieff and N.R. Lieff (Eds.), *The psychological basis for medical practice*. New York: Harper & Rowe.

Lingard, L. (2009). What we see and don't see when we look at 'competence': notes on a god term. *Advances in Health Sciences Education Theory and Practice*.14(5) 625-8.

Lingard, L., Reznick, R. (2002). Forming professional identities on a health care team: discursive construction of the 'other' in the operating room.*Medical Education,* 36,728-34..

Luhrmann, T. M. (2000). *Of two minds: An anthropologist looks at American Psychiatry*. New York, NY: Vintage Books.

Lutz, C. (2007). Emotion, Thought and Estrangement: Emotion as a Cultural Category. In Helena Wulff(ed.), *The Emotions: A Cultural Reader* 19-29. Oxford, UK, New York, NY: Berg publishing.

Lutz, C. (1988). *Unnatural emotions*. Chicago: University of Chicago Press.

Lutz, C., Abu-Lughod, L. (1990). Introduction: Emotion, discourse and the politics of everyday life. In C.A. Lutz & L. Abu-Lughod (Eds.), *Language and the politics of emotion*. Cambridge, UK: Cambridge University Press.

Lutz, C., White, G. (1996). The Anthropology of emotions.*Annual.Review.Of Anthropology.* 15, 405-436.

Magellsen, S. (2009)."Theatre immersion" and the simulation of theatres of war.*TDR: The Drama Review,* 53(1), 47-71.

Magnusson, J. (2011). Academic activism and nomadic paths.InJ.Newson& C. Polster (Eds.), *Academic callings* 153-162. Toronto, ON: Canadian Scholar's Press Inc.

Martimianakis, M., Manaiate, J., Hodges, B. (2009).Sociological interpretations of professionalism.*Medical Education,* 43: 829-837.

Massumi, B. (2002a). Introduction, Like a Thought. In *A Shock to Thought: Expression after deleuze and guattari*. London and New York: Routledge Press

Massumi, B. (2002b). Introduction, Concrete is as concrete doesn't. In *Parables of the virtual: Movement, affect, sensation*. Durham & London, UK: Duke University Press.

Matsumoto, E., Hamstra, S., Radomski, S., Cusimano, M. (2002).The effect of bench model fidelity on endourological skills: a randomized controlled study. *The Journal of Urology,* 167(3), 1243-47.

McConachie, B. (2007). Falsifiable theories for theatre and performance studies.*Theatre Journal.*59.553-577.

McLaren, P. (1996). Liberatory politics and higher education: A Freirean perspective. In: H. Giroux, C. Lankshear, P. McLaren & M. Peters (Eds.), *Counternarratives: Cultural Studies and Critical Pedagogies in Postmodern Spaces* 117-147. London: Routledge.

McNaughton, N, Tiberius, R. (1999).The effects of portraying psychologically and emotionally complex standardized patient roles. *Teaching and Learning in Medicine,* 11,135-141.

McNaughton, N. (2003). *Standardized patient's experiences of long psychiatry exam stations: A case study.* Unpublished Master's Thesis. Ontario Institute for Studies in Education, Toronto, ON: University of Toronto.

McNaughton, N. (2008a) Where is the patient in the standardized patient? Published Abstract, *International Ottawa Conference on Medical Education*: Melbourne, Australia.

McNaughton, N., Ravitz, P., Waddell, A., Hodges, B. (2008a). Psychiatric education and simulation: A review of the literature. *Canadian Journal of Psychiatry, 53(2), 85-93.*

McWhinney, I. (2003). The evolution of the clinical method. In M. Stewart, W. Weston, I. McWhinney, (Eds.), *Patient centred medicine: Transforming the clinical method, (second ed.)* (p.17-30). Oxford, UK: Radcliffe Medical Press.

Mesko, B., Ann Myers Medical Center: the future of medical education website. Retrieved on November 20, 2010.http://ammc.wordpress.com/2007/06/01the-beginning;2007.

Micale, M. (Ed.).(2004).*The mind of modernism.*Stanford CA: Stanford Press.

Mills, S. (1997/2004). *Discourse: the new critical idiom.* New York, NY: Routledge.

Murrell, J. (1977). *Waiting for the parade.* Toronto, ON: Samuel French Inc.

Myers, B.W., Alexander, B.K. (2010). (Performance Is) Metaphor as a methodological tool in qualitative inquiry. *International review of qualitative research*, 3 (2), 163-171.

Nelles, L.J. (2011). My body, their stories. *Canadian Theatre review (CTR).* 146:55-61.

Neufeld, V., Maudsley, R., Pickering, R., Turnbull, J., Weston, W., Brown, M., Simpson, J. (1998). Educating Future Physicians for Ontario. *Academic Medicine,* 73, (11), 1133-1148.

Newman, F., Holzman, L. (1997). *The end of knowing: A new developmental way of learning.* London, UK: Routledge.

Noddings, N. (1984). *Caring, a feminine approach to ethics & moral education.* Berkeley, CA: University of California Press.

Norman, G.R., Van der Vleuten, C.P.M., Irby, D.I. (Eds). (2002). Assessment of non-cognitive factors. In *International handbook of research in medical education. (p.* 711-755). Dordrecht, the Netherlands: Kluwer Academic Publishers.

Norman, G.R., Barrows, H.S., Gliva, G., Woodward, C.A. (1985). Simulated patients. InV.R. Neufeld, G.R. Norman, (Eds.). *Assessing clinical competence* (p. 219-229). New York, NY: Springer-Verla.

Norman, G R. (1999). The Adult learner: A mythical species. *Academic Medicine*, 74(8), 886-888.

Nussbaum, M. (1996).Compassion: The Basic social emotion. *Social Philosophy and Policy*, 13(1), 27-58.

O'Riley, P. (2003). *Technology, culture, and socioeconomics: A rhizoanalysis of educational discourses.*NewYork, Washington, DC, Bern, Oxford: Peter Lang.

Orner, M. (1992).Interrupting the calls for student voice in "Liberatory" education: A feminist post structuralist perspective. In C. Luke, J. Gore, (Eds.), *Feminisms and critical pedagogy. (p. 74-90).* New York, NY, London, UK: Routledge.

Payne, W.L. (1983/1986). A Study of emotion, developing emotional intelligence: self integration relating to fear, pain and desire. *Dissertation Abstracts International, 47,* 203A. (University microfilms No. AAC 8605928).

Percival, T. (1927).*Medical ethics: or, a code of institutes and precept, adapted to the professional conduct of physicians and surgeons.* (Third Ed.), London, UK: Oxford Press (retrieved through Google books online).

Phillips, N., Hardy, C. (2002). *Discourse analysis: Investigating processes of social construction.* London, New York. Sage Publications.

Plato "The Republic".In T. Cole. H.K. Chinoy, (Eds.), (1970). *Actors on acting: The theories, techniques and practices of the world's great actors.* (p. 6 -11). New York, NY:Three Rivers Press.

Porter, R. (1993). The Body and the Mind, the Doctor and the Patient: Negotiating Hysteria. In S. Gilman (Ed.), *Hysteria beyond Freud.*(p. 225-

285). Berkeley, CA, Los Angeles, CA, London, UK: University of California Press.

Prideaux, D., Bligh, J. (2002). Research in medical education: asking the right questions. *Medical Education,* 36 (12), 1114–1115.

Rabinow, P. (1984). *The Foucault Reader.* New York, NY: Random House.

Rabow, M., Reman, R., Parmelee, D., Innui, T. (2010). Professional formation: Extending medicine's lineage of service into the next century. *Academic Medicine,* 85(2), 310-317.

Reeves, S., Fox, A., Hodges, B. (2009). The Competence movement in the health professions: Ensuring consistent standards or reproducing conventional domains of practice? *Advances in Health Sciences Education Theory and Practice,* 14(4), 451-3.

Reinelt, J., Roach, J., (Eds) (2007/2010). *Critical theory and performance* (Second Ed.).Ann Arbor Michigan: University of Michigan Press.

Roach, J. (1985).*The Player's passion: Studies in the science of acting.* Ann Arbor, Michigan: The University of Michigan Press.

Robinson, K. (2003). The passion and the pleasure: Foucault's art of not being oneself. *Theory, Culture & Society,* 20(2), 119-144.

Rose, N., (1985). *The Psychological complex: Psychology, politics and society in England 1869-1939.* London, UK, Boston, MA, Melbourne, Australia: Routledge&Kegan Paul.

Rose, N. (1990). Governing the soul: the shaping of the private self. London, UK, New York, NY: Routledge.

Rose, N. (1998). *Inventing ourselves: Psychology, power and personhood.* Cambridge U.K: University Press.

Rosen, K.R. (2008). The history of medical simulation.*Journal of Critical Care,* 23, 157-166.

Salovey, P., Mayer, J.D. (1990). Emotional Intelligence.*Imagination, Cognition, and Personality*; 9,185-211.

Salovey, P., Grewal, D. (2005). The Science of Emotional intelligence.*Current Directions in Psychological Sciences,* 14, 281-285.

Satterfield, J., Hughes, E. (2007). Emotion skills training for medical students: a systematic review. *Medical Education,* 41, 935-941.

Scott, J. (1991). The evidence of experience.*Critical Inquiry, 17(4),* 773-797.

Shildrick, M. (2002).*Embodying the monster: Encounters with the vulnerable self.* London, UK, Thousand Oaks, CA: Sage Publications.

Shirley, J., Padgett, S. (2006). An analysis of the discourse of professionalism. In D. Wear, J. Aultman(Eds.), *Professionalism in Medicine: Critical Perspectives*. (p.25-43). New York, NY: Springer.

Showalter, E. (1993). Hysteria, feminism and gender.In, Gilman S. (Ed.).*Hysteria beyond Freud.*(p.286-344). Berkeley, CA, Los Angeles, CA, London, UK: University of California Press

Simpson, M., Buckman, R., Stewart, M, Maguire, P., Lipkin, M., Novack ,D., Till, J. (1991). Doctor-patient communication: the Toronto consensus statement. *British Medical Journal,* 303, 1385-87.

Sinclair, S. (1997). *Making doctors: An institutional apprenticeship.* Oxford, UK, NewYork, NY: Berg Publishing.

Smith, A., Kleinman, S. (1989). Managing emotions in medical school: Students' contacts with the living and the dead. *Social Psychology Quarterly,* 52(1), 56-69.

South, R. (1688). A Sermon Delivered at Christ-Church, Oxon., Before the University, Octob. 14. 1688: Prov. XII.22 Lying Lips are abomination to the Lord", pp. 519–657 in South, R., *Twelve Sermons Preached Upon Several Occasions* (Second Edition), Volume I, Printed by S.D. for Thomas Bennet, (London), 1697. Retrieved September 2010.http://en.wikipedia.org/wiki/Simulation.

Spelman, E. (1997). *Fruits of sorrow: Framing our attention to suffering.* Boston: Beacon Press.

Spencer, H. (1862). *First principles.*London, UK: Williams &Norgate.

Spencer, J. (2004). Decline in empathy in medical education: How can we stop the Rot? *Medical Education,* 38(9), 916-918.

Stanislavski, C, (1936). *An actor prepares.* (E. R. Hapgood, Trans.). New York, NY: Theatre Arts Books.

Starr, P. (1982). *The social transformation of American medicine.*U.S.A: Basic Books.

Stepien, K, Baernstein A. (2006). Educating for empathy.*Journal of General Internal Medicine, 21*, 524-530.

Szasz, T. (1996).*The Meaning of mind: Language, morality, and neuroscience.* Westport, CT, London, UK: Praeger.

Tamboukou, M. (1999).Writing genealogies: an exploration of Foucault's strategies for doing research.*Discourse Studies in the Cultural politics of Education.* Vol. 20, Issue 2, pages 201 – 217.

Tamboukou, M. (2003).Interrogating the 'emotional turn': making connections with Foucault and Deleuze.*European Journal of Counseling and Health,6(3)*, 209-223.

Tassi, A. (2000). Performance as metamorphosis.*Consciousness, Literature and the Arts.*1(2), 1 – 20.

Taylor, C. (1989). *Sources of the self: The making of modern Identity.* Cambridge, MA: Harvard University Press.

Taylor, J. (2011). The moral aesthetics of simulated suffering in standardized patient performances.*Culture, Medicine and Psychiatry, 35(2), 134-162.doi:* 10.1007/s11013-011-9211-5.

Toumlins, S. (1992). *Cosmopolis: the hidden agenda of modernity.* Chicago, IL: University of Chicago Press.

Van der Vleuten, C.P.M., Swanson, D.B. (1990). Assessment of clinical skills with standardized patients; State of the art.*Teaching and Learning in Medicine*, 2, 58-76.

Vu, N.V., Barrows, H.S. (1994). Use of standardized patients in clinical assessments: Recent developments and measurement findings. *Educational Researcher*; 23, 23-30.

Wallace, P. (1997). Following the threads of an innovation: The history of standardized patients in medical education, *Caduceus.* Autumn,3(13) 5-28.

Weber, F.P. (1911). On the association of hysteria and malingering and on the phylogenetic aspect of Hysteria as pathological exaggeration (or disorder) of tertiary (nervous) sex characters.*Association of Hysteria and Malingering.*26-36.

Wear, D., Varley, J. (2008). Rituals of verification: the role of simulation in developing and evaluating empathic communication. *Patient Education and Counseling.*7, 153-156

Wear, D., Aultman, J. (2006). D. Wear, J. Aultman, (Eds.), *Professionalism in medicine: critical perspectives.* New York, NY: Springer.

Wear, D. (1997). *Privilege in the medical academy: A feminist examines gender, race and power.* New York, NY, London, UK: Teachers College Press.

Whitehead, C. (2010). Recipes for medical education reform: Will different ingredients create better doctors? A commentary on Sales and Schaff.*Social Science and Medicine,* 70, 1680 -1685.

Williams, S. (2001). *Emotion and social theory.* London, UK: Sage.

Woodward, K. (2009). *Statistical panic: Cultural politics and poetics of the emotions.* Durham, UK, London, UK: Duke University Press.

Wulff, H. (2007). (Ed.) *The emotions: A cultural reader* Oxford, UK, New York, NY: Berg publishing

Yeatman, A. (1994). Postmodern epistemological politics and social science. In Gloria Anzaldua (Ed.), *Making face, making soul: Creative and critical perspectives by feminists of color* 187-202. London, UK: Routledge.

Yee, B., Naik, V.N., Joo, H.S., Savoldelli, G.L., Chung, D.Y., Houston, P.L., Karatzoglou, B.J., Haemstra, S.J. (2005). Nontechnical skills in anaesthesia crisis management with repeated exposure to simulation-based education, *Anesthesiology,* 103(2), 241-248.

Zembylas, M. (2007). Risks and pleasures: a Deleuzo-Guattarian pedagogy of desire in education. *British Educational Research Journal,* 33(3), 331-347.

Zembylas, M. (2005). Teaching with emotion: A postmodern enactment. Greenwich CT: InformationAge Publishing.

Zournazi, M. (2002).Navigating movements: An interview with Brian Massumi.Retrieved June 2010.http://www.21cmagazine.com/issue2/massumi.html

MoreBooks! publishing

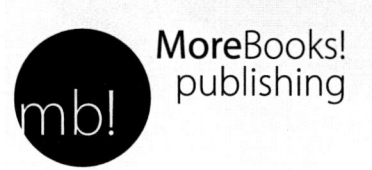

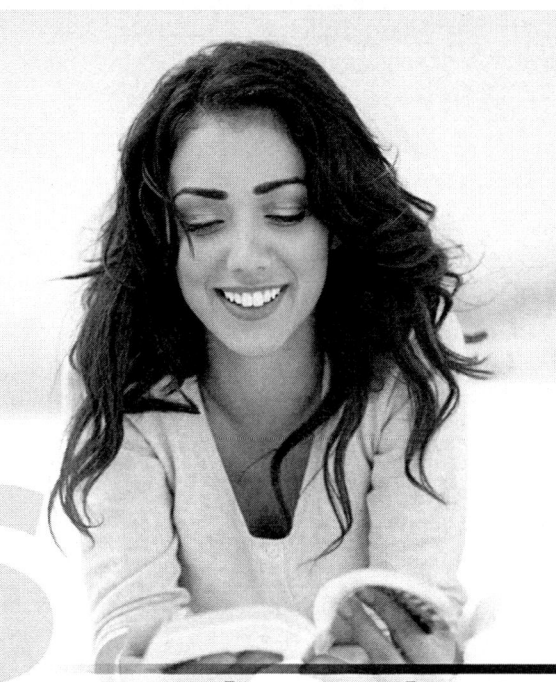

i want morebooks!

Buy your books fast and straightforward online - at one of world's fastest growing online book stores! Environmentally sound due to Print-on-Demand technologies.

Buy your books online at
www.get-morebooks.com

Kaufen Sie Ihre Bücher schnell und unkompliziert online – auf einer der am schnellsten wachsenden Buchhandelsplattformen weltweit! Dank Print-On-Demand umwelt- und ressourcenschonend produziert.

Bücher schneller online kaufen
www.morebooks.de

VDM Verlagsservicegesellschaft mbH
Heinrich-Böcking-Str. 6-8　　Telefon: +49 681 3720 174　　info@vdm-vsg.de
D - 66121 Saarbrücken　　　Telefax: +49 681 3720 1749　　www.vdm-vsg.de

Printed by
Schaltungsdienst Lange o.H.G., Berlin